TALKABOUT TRANSITIONS

This is a comprehensive programme of activities designed to support young people as they make the transition from education to employment. Following the hugely successful *TALKABOUT* structure, the programme is broken down into topics and activities, each constructed to teach the skills necessary for further education or employment. Topics explore the various opportunities available to school leavers, offer guidance on the application and interview processes and consider the skills necessary to make employment a success. Exploring transition as a process of discovery, this programme takes the fear and uncertainty out of this time of change.

The resource includes:

- Assessment and evaluation forms to help assess the needs of the individual and personalise the programme
- 40 engaging activities
- Fully photocopiable and downloadable colour resources to facilitate group sessions

This book is an invaluable resource for professionals working with teenagers and young adults with SEMH needs, autism spectrum disorders and intellectual disabilities. The programme would also benefit teenagers and young people daunted by change or struggling to find or remain in employment.

Chris Mcloughlin graduated from the University of East Anglia in 2011 with a BSc (Hons) in *Speech and Language Therapy* and joined Alex Kelly Ltd in 2013. He has gained a wide variety of experience, working and training in mainstream, special and SEMH schools and colleges, and he now specialises in working with people with intellectual disabilities and autism. He is also the manager of the therapy department at Speaking Space Ltd.

Alex Kelly is a speech and language therapist with over 30 years' experience of working with both children and adults with an intellectual disability (learning disability) and specialising in working with people who have difficulties with social skills. She runs her own businesses (Alex Kelly Ltd and Speaking Space Ltd) with her husband Brian Sains and is the author of a number of books and resources, including the best-selling *TALKABOUT* series.

She is based in Hampshire, in the south of England. Alex Kelly Ltd provides training and consultancy work to schools and organisations in social skills, self-esteem and relationship skills around the UK and abroad. Speaking Space Ltd also provides speech and language therapy in a number of schools in and around Hampshire, training in all aspects of autism and communication, and a Total Communication day service for adults with an intellectual disability or autism. In 2019 Speaking Space Ltd was Autism Accredited by the National Autistic Society with advanced status.

You can contact Alex or Chris through the website **www.speakingspace.co.uk.**

MORE BRILLIANT PROFESSIONAL RESOURCES FROM BESTSELLING AUTHOR ALEX KELLY!

TALKABOUT

Each practical workbook in this bestselling series provides a clear programme of activities designed to improve self-awareness, self-esteem and social skills.

'All in all, Alex, what a wonderful world for kids it would be if your social skills programme were in all schools across the continents' – Catherine Varapodio Longley, Parent, Melbourne, 2013.

'I feel very lucky to work in a school where our pupils get the opportunity to utilise Talkabout resources and to see the benefit that this has made to them and their peers. You are making a difference!' – Nicole Thomas, Teacher, 2017

Title	Focus	Age range
Talkabout (2nd edition)	Developing social skills for all ages	7+
Talkabout for Children 1 (2nd edition)	Developing self-awareness and self-esteem	4–11
Talkabout for Children 2 (2nd edition)	Developing social skills	4–11
Talkabout for Children 3 (2nd edition)	Developing friendship skills	4–11
Talkabout for Teenagers (2nd edition)	Developing social and emotional communication skills	11–19
Talkabout Transitions	Moving from education to employment	16+
Talkabout for Adults	Developing self-awareness and self-esteem in adults	16+
Talkabout Relationships	Developing relationship skills	11+
Talkabout Sex and Relationships 1	Developing intimate relationship skills	11+
Talkabout Sex and Relationships 2	Sex education	11+
Talkabout Assessment	Social skills assessment tool	7+
Talkabout DVD	Developing social skills	7+
Talkabout Board Game	Developing social communication skills, self-esteem and friendship skills	7+
Talkabout Cards: Group Cohesion Games	Group cohesion	7+
Talkabout Cards: Self Awareness Activities	Developing self-awareness	7+

TALKABOUT TRANSITIONS

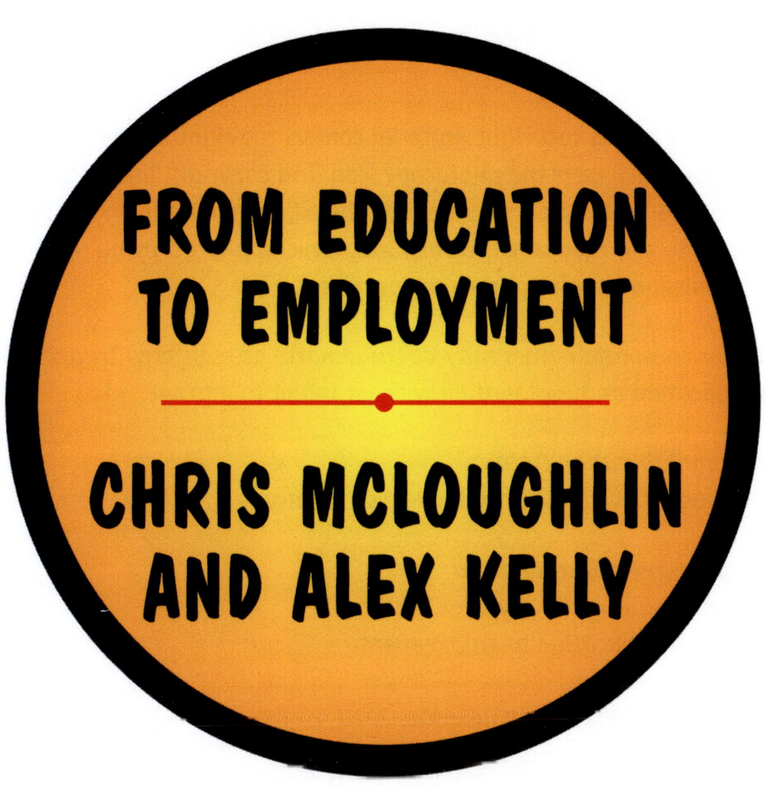

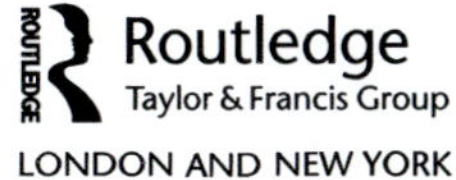

Routledge
Taylor & Francis Group

LONDON AND NEW YORK

First published 2020
by Routledge
2 Park Square, Milton Park, Abingdon, Oxon OX14 4RN

and by Routledge
52 Vanderbilt Avenue, New York, NY 10017

Routledge is an imprint of the Taylor & Francis Group, an informa business

British Library Cataloguing-in-Publication Data
A catalogue record for this book is available from the British Library

Library of Congress Cataloging-in-Publication Data
Names: Mcloughlin, Christopher, author. | Kelly, Alex, author.
Title: Talkabout transitions : from education to employment /
    Christopher Mcloughlin and Alex Kelly.
Description: Abingdon, Oxon ; New York, NY : Routledge, 2020. |
    Includes bibliographical references and index.
Identifiers: LCCN 2019025095 (print) | LCCN 2019025096 (ebook) |
    ISBN 9781138606890 (paperback) | ISBN 9780429467448 (ebook)
Subjects: LCSH: School-to-work transition. | High school students—
    Vocational guidance. | Students with disabilities—Vocational guidance.
Classification: LCC LC1037 .M45 2020 (print) | LCC LC1037 (ebook) |
    DDC 371.19/5—dc23
LC record available at https://lccn.loc.gov/2019025095
LC ebook record available at https://lccn.loc.gov/2019025096

ISBN: 978-1-138-60689-0 (pbk)
ISBN: 978-0-429-46744-8 (ebk)

Typeset in ITC Flora
by Apex CoVantage, LLC

Visit the companion website: www.routledge.com/cw/kelly 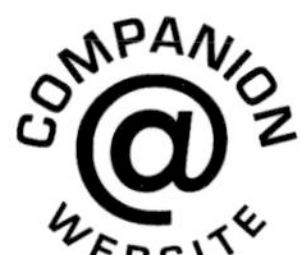

Contents   Page

Acknowledgements

Chris: I'd like to thank my wife, Katie Andrews, for supporting me in everything I try at home and in work.

Alex: I'd like to thank my husband Brian Sains and our boys, Ed, Pete and George.

We'd both like to mention our colleagues, who are all brilliant: Joley Anderson, Grace Anstey, Ali Banham, Lauren Bush, Marnie Daws, Megan Evans, Abby Goodrich, Natalie Hamilton, Ellie Jones, Amy Keable, Pete Kelly, Abbie Michael, Marleen Mohanlol, Alec Morley, Deborah Niblett, Naomi Pearson, Marina Trivett, Emily Tully, Anne Waggott. We would especially like to thank Amy Green, Katherine Wareham and Zara Baillie for trialling the programme and providing helpful feedback.

About the authors

Chris Mcloughlin graduated from the University of East Anglia in 2011 with a BSc (Hons) in Speech and Language Therapy and joined Alex Kelly Ltd in 2013. He has gained a wide variety of experience, working and training in mainstream, special and SEMH schools and colleges, and he now specialises in working with people with intellectual disabilities and autism. He is also the manager of the therapy department at Speaking Space Ltd.

Alex Kelly is a speech and language therapist with over 30 years' experience of working with both children and adults with an intellectual disability (learning disability) and specialising in working with people who have difficulties with social skills. She runs her own businesses (Alex Kelly Ltd and Speaking Space Ltd) with her husband Brian Sains and is the author of a number of books and resources, including the best-selling TALKABOUT series.

She is based in Hampshire, in the south of England. Alex Kelly Ltd provides training and consultancy work to schools and organisations in social skills, self-esteem and relationship skills around the UK and abroad. Speaking Space Ltd also provides speech and language therapy in a number of schools in and around Hampshire, training in all aspects of autism and communication, and a Total Communication day service for adults with an intellectual disability or autism. In 2019 Speaking Space Ltd was Autism Accredited by the National Autistic Society with advanced status.

You can contact Alex or Chris through the website **www.speakingspace.co.uk.**

🕴 Introduction

The theory behind the book

When young people move on from school or college and start the transition to becoming an adult, there are many changes that take place. They are developing friendships and intimate relationships, managing their own time, money and behaviour, and thinking about further education and possible careers (Clark & Unruh, 2009).

Being in employment is important for most of us throughout our lives and not only because it means that we have a source of income to spend on hobbies, holidays and supporting ourselves and our family. Meaningful employment provides us with a sense of belonging, contributes to having positive self-esteem and provides us with an environment to build workplace relationships. Having a job has been shown to have a positive impact on both our physical and mental health (Waddell & Burton, 2006), whereas those in long-term unemployment are more likely to experience depression, anxiety and poorer physical health (National Mental Health Development Unit, 2010). There is also evidence to suggest that participating in further or higher education leads to increased employment opportunities and increased pay, as well as better self-esteem and well-being (Department for Business, Innovation and Skills, 2013).

There are many routes to gaining employment and it's important that those responsible for young people of transition age lay out the available options (Clark & Unruh, 2009), as 'if there are no real choices about future destinations then any transition process is doomed before it begins' (Broadhurst et al., 2012). This book explores the routes available to most young people, including employment, further and higher education, apprenticeships, work experience and/or volunteering and ensures that young people participating in the programme can complete a CV and application forms.

Whilst at school and college, young people often develop the technical skills needed to gain employment, like reading, writing and maths, but often it is their soft skills which are most useful in supporting them to find and keep employment (Robles, 2012). Soft skills are the personal qualities we have when working with others, including communication and social skills, problem-solving, time-management and professionalism, amongst others. These skills are important to show to employers during the interview process (Schulz, 2008). Having good soft skills also allows us to work in a team successfully (Nickson et al., 2011), developing positive and harmonious relationships with our colleagues along the way.

Facilitators using this resource with a group of young people should see the work around transitions as a 'period of "discovery"' (Clark & Unruh, 2009) and 'a process, not an event'

(Broadhurst et al., 2012). The group leaders should foster a person-centred approach, focusing on possible aims and outcomes for the future of the young person, whilst building on their specific strengths and problem-solving skills to ensure they are successful (Clark & Unruh, 2009). If we can do this for all young people moving on to adulthood, whilst encouraging the development of transferable soft skills, this will provide the greatest opportunity to thrive and succeed.

An overview of the book

TALKABOUT TRANSITIONS is a practical and structured resource that has been designed to support therapists and teaching staff to teach the skills necessary for employment or further education. Each topic builds on the previous one and has activities and worksheets that focus on the relevant skills.

The activities in this book are designed for working with people in groups but can be adapted for working on a one-to-one basis.

TALKABOUT TRANSITIONS is divided into six topics.

Assessment
This includes a one-to-one interview to provide a baseline score to measure progress.

Topic 1 – This is me
This topic helps the group get to know each other using activities that focus on self-awareness, self-esteem and group gelling.

Topic 2 – Which route do I take?
This topic explores the different employment and education options that the group have available, including activities around jobs, education and local institutions.

Topic 3 – Application process
This topic explores the different ways that group members can apply for jobs, including CVs, covering letters, application forms and personal statements.

Topic 4 – Interviews
This topic aims to develop the interview skills of the group members, through activities focusing on body language, the way we talk and answering common interview questions.

Topic 5 – Workplace relationships
This topic aims to support the group members to develop effective workplace relationships, including activities on small talk, dealing with conflict and working in a team.

Topic 6 – Problem-solving

This topic is optional but recommended. The activities in this topic are soft skills that
are important to develop for work and adult life but are not directly related to employment
or further education. It is important to complete the rest of the topics before this one,
but it may be possible to pick and choose certain activities if tackling an issue within
the group. This topic aims to develop the group members' problem-solving skills and
ability to reflect through a variety of frameworks, as well as provide a structure for time-
management.

Who is *TALKABOUT TRANSITIONS* aimed at?

This resource is primarily aimed at teenagers or adults who are leaving secondary school,
college or sixth form within the next year or two. The programme was piloted in schools,
colleges and sixth forms for teenagers with social, emotional and mental health (SEMH) needs,
autism spectrum disorders and mild learning disabilities. It is also felt that some teenagers
who are leaving mainstream school, college or sixth form would benefit from the practical
activities available in this book. This book may also benefit young adults who are unsuccessful
in obtaining or remaining in employment.

When considering if someone is suitable for this programme, it may help to ask the following
questions:

- Are they unsure of where they will be going after the academic year finishes?
- Are they unsure what career they would like to do when they leave education?
- Are they unsure of how to apply for jobs or further education?
- Do they lack confidence in interviews?
- Do they struggle to make and maintain positive relationships?
- Do they struggle with solving problems in a timely and effective way?

The person should also have the following skills:

- Good self-awareness
- An ability to express themselves adequately in a group setting
- An ability to work within a group setting
- Motivation to attend a group

Setting up and running a TALKABOUT group

Group membership

It is important to match the group members in terms of their needs and how well they are
going to get on. A group is far more likely to gel and work well if they have similar needs, are

a similar age and like each other. Group membership should also be closed, i.e. you should not allow new members to join half way through as this will alter the group dynamics.

The size of the group

Groups work best if they are not too small or too big, preferably between four and eight. Six group members is ideal. You need the group to be small enough to make sure that everyone contributes and feels part of the group and large enough to make activities such as role plays and group discussions feasible and interesting. Even numbers are helpful if you are going to ask them to sometimes work in pairs.

Whilst it is recommended that this book be used with a small group, it may be that the activities and worksheets are relevant for a larger class. If appropriate, split the class into smaller groups or pairs to complete the activities and encourage feedback at the end. It is still recommended that teaching staff adhere to the structure of a Talkabout group, but this may differ in a school environment.

Length of the group

Timings are given at the beginning of each topic. In terms of the sessions, it is important that you have enough time to get through your session plan (see next section) but not so much time that the group members get bored. 40–45 minutes would be appropriate.

Group leaders

Groups run better with two leaders, especially as there is often a need to model behaviours, observe the group members, work video cameras and facilitate group discussions.

Accommodation

You will need a room that is comfortable for the group members to learn in where you are not going to be interrupted. Don't be tempted to accept the corner of the hall or library as an acceptable place to run your group – this will not help your group members to relax and talk openly. In terms of the layout of chairs, it is sometimes preferable to work around a table depending on the activity.

Cohesiveness

A group that does not gel will not learn or have fun. It is therefore important to take time to ensure that group gelling occurs. Things that help are:

- interpersonal attraction – people who like each other are more likely to gel
- people who have similar needs
- activities that encourage everyone to take part and have fun
- arrange the chairs into a circle prior to the group
- ensure that everyone feels valued in the group

- ensure that everyone feels part of the group and has an equal 'say'
- ask the group to set some rules
- start each session with a simple activity that is fun and stress-free
- finish each session with another activity that is fun and stress-free

The format of the session

The format of the session will vary from time to time but there are general guidelines which should be followed:

1 Group cohesion activity

This is an essential part of the group. It brings the group together and helps them to focus on the other group members and the purpose of the group. The activity should be simple, stress-free and involve all.

2 How are you feeling?

This should be done every session to ensure children learn how to express their feelings and for the facilitator to address any concerns. There is a feelings board in Topic 1 of this book.

3 Main activity(s)

This will include the activity that you are facilitating from the Transitions programme. It is during this part of the session that it is most important not to lose people's attention by allowing an activity to go on for too long, or one person to dominate the conversation.

4 Finishing activity

Each session should end with a group activity to bring the group back together again and to reduce anxiety if the clients have found any of the activities difficult. The activity should therefore be fun, simple and stress-free.

How *TALKABOUT TRANSITIONS* works with other *TALKABOUT* resources

The ideas and activities throughout this book draw on a wide variety of social skills that have been described and developed in other Talkabout books. If you feel that the group you are working with don't have the requisite skills in a certain area of the social skills hierarchy, it is worth looking back at previous Talkabout books to focus on these skills in more depth. *Talkabout (2nd Edition): A Social Communication Package* and *Talkabout for Teenagers: Developing Social and Emotional Communication Skills* are the recommended additional reading as these focus on the core skills of self-awareness, self-esteem and social skills targeted at adolescents and young adults.

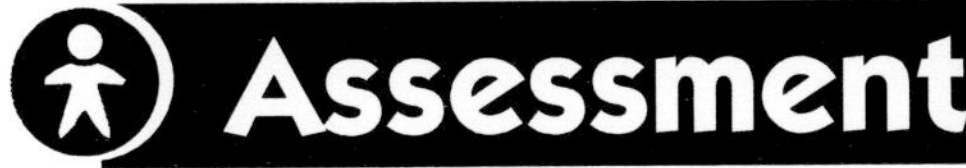

Assessment

Objectives

To provide an overview of the group member's understanding of their own qualities, skills and interests, as well as their awareness of qualifications, employment and interviews. It can also help you to see how the group member responds to problems at home and at school/college.

Timing

This depends on how well you know the group member but it will take up to 30 minutes.

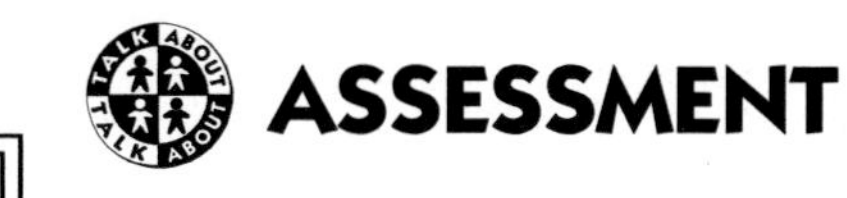 **ASSESSMENT**

Transitions interview

Name: .... DoB: ....

Class: .... Date: ....

Instructions: Sit somewhere calm and quiet. Explain that you would like to ask a few questions to get to know the group member better. Let them know that it's fine if they're not sure of the answer or don't want to answer a question.

1. Tell me about yourself. *What are your interests? What are you like?*
2. What do you like doing? What are you good at? *At home? At school/college?*
3. What do you dislike? What do you find difficult? *At home? At school/college?*
4. What do you want to do when you leave school/college?

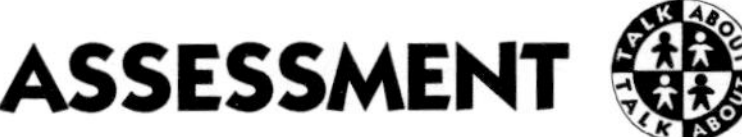

5. What skills/qualifications do you need to be able to do... (use answer from above)?

6. What different things could you do when you leave school/college?
e.g. university/apprenticeship/volunteering/job

7. Have you been to an interview before? What happens at an interview?

8. What do you do when you have a problem?
In school/college?

Outside of school/college?

Summary and comments:

Completed by: .... Date: ....

ASSESSMENT

Topic 1 – This is me

Objectives
To develop a cohesive group through activities that focus on aspects of self-awareness and self-esteem.

To introduce the topic of transition and what this might mean for the individuals leaving their current provision.

To start considering qualities and interests that are relevant to future employment or education.

Timing
This topic will take up to six sessions to complete.

Activity	Description
How am I feeling? (Activity 1)	*Pass the feelings board around the group and find out how everyone is feeling and, if they would like to share, find out why.*
Who am I? (Activity 2)	*The group members take it in turns to turn over the cards and share something about themselves.*
Where am I? (Activity 3)	*Group members explore the geography of their country in a movement game and find their location on a map.*
Useful qualities (Activity 4)	*The group is asked to discuss what qualities would be useful and not useful for certain jobs.*
My qualities (Activity 5)	*The group members decide what their useful qualities are and think about one quality they could work on.*
What do I like to do? (Activity 6)	*The group members think about their favourite interest, hobby or lesson, and what skills and qualities they need to carry it out well.*
Advertise me (Activity 7)	*Group members create an advert summary of all their interests, skills and qualities.*

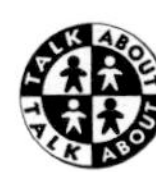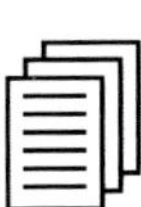

Activity 1 How am I feeling?

Preparation

Print out and laminate the feelings board you wish to use. One board has 19 emotions and the other has 15. Both have a question mark for 'other'. If you feel your group needs a simpler board you could refer to *Talkabout for Adults* or *Talkabout for Children 1 (2nd edition): Developing Self-Awareness and Self-Esteem* for more choices.

Instructions

- Introduce the emotions and the facial expressions.

- Pass the board around the group members and ask them to say how they are feeling. Encourage them to ask each other.

- Can they share with the group why they are feeling that way?

- The '?' is for people to choose another emotion that is not on the board, for example they may be feeling 'hungry' or 'lonely'.

- This works well as a starter activity for each session.

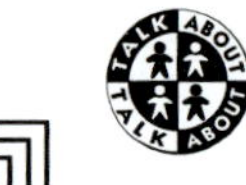

Activity 1 How am I feeling?

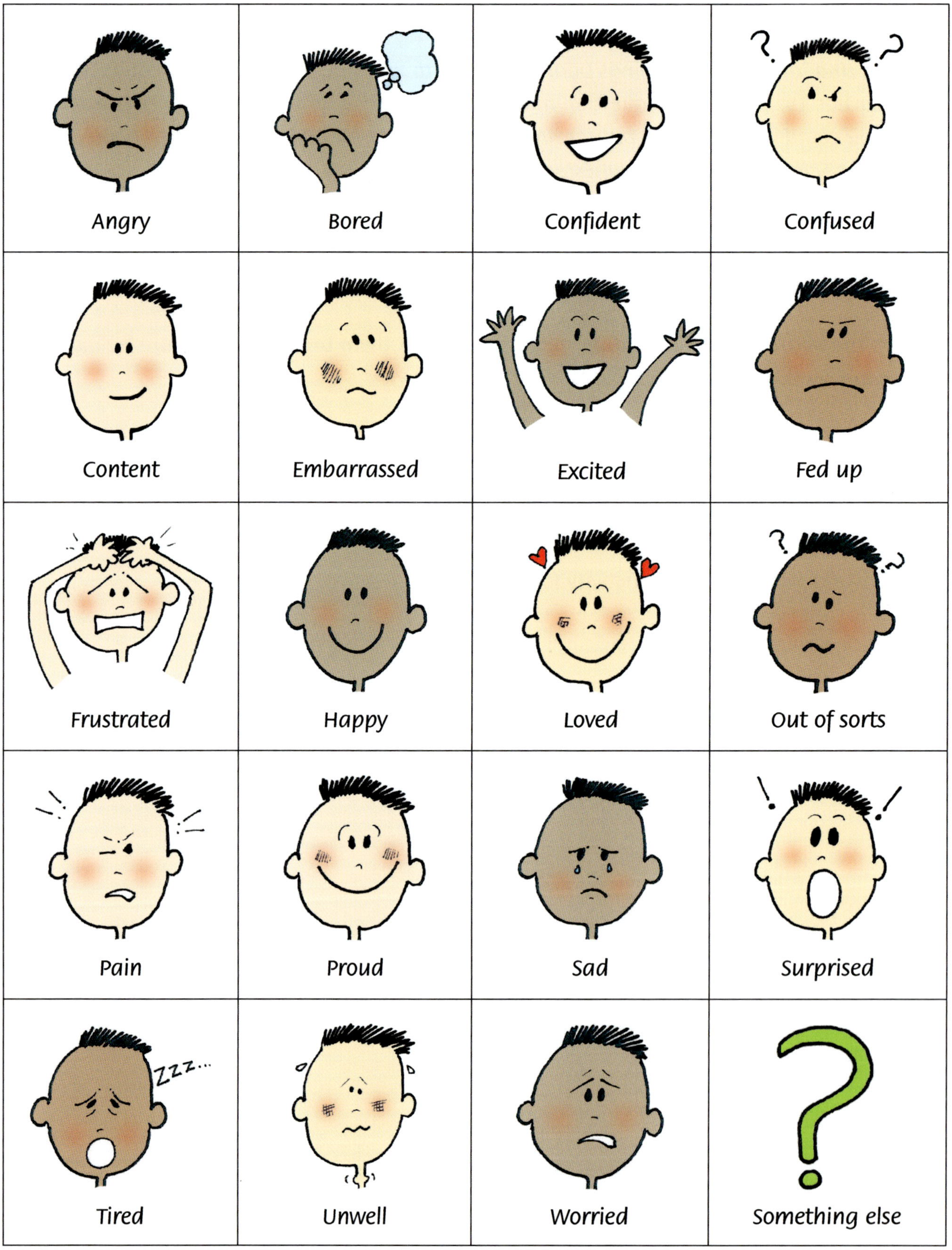

Angry	Bored	Confident	Confused
Content	Embarrassed	Excited	Fed up
Frustrated	Happy	Loved	Out of sorts
Pain	Proud	Sad	Surprised
Tired	Unwell	Worried	Something else

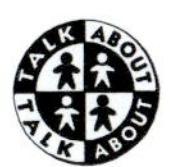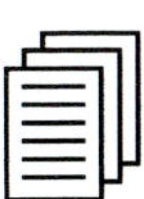

Activity 1 How am I feeling?

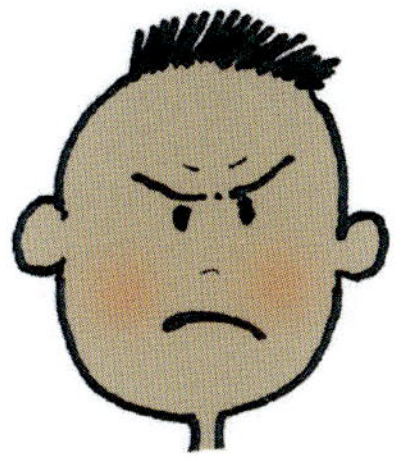 Angry	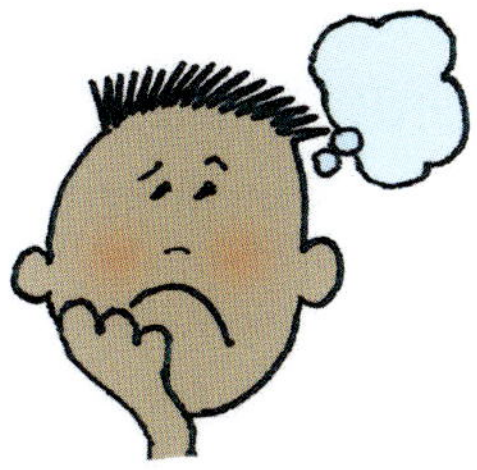 Bored	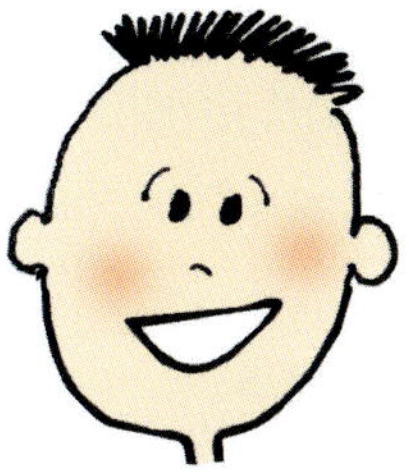 Confident
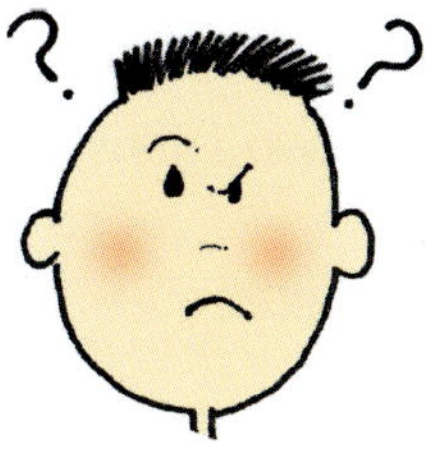 Confused	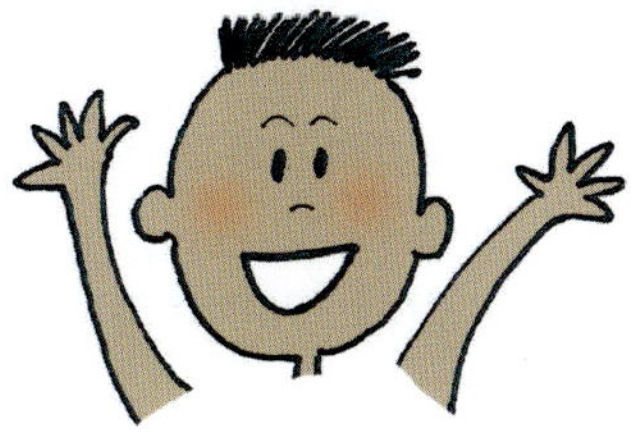 Excited	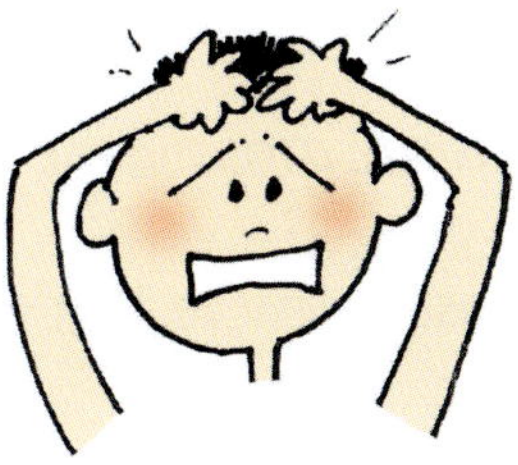 Frustrated
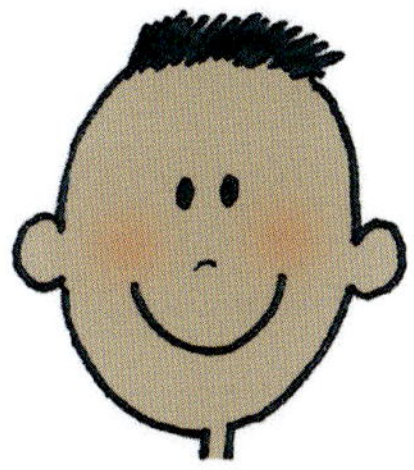 Happy	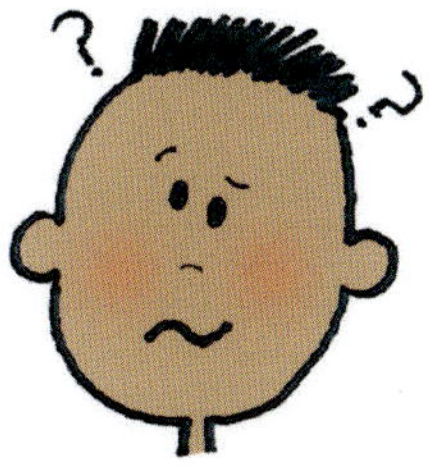 Out of sorts	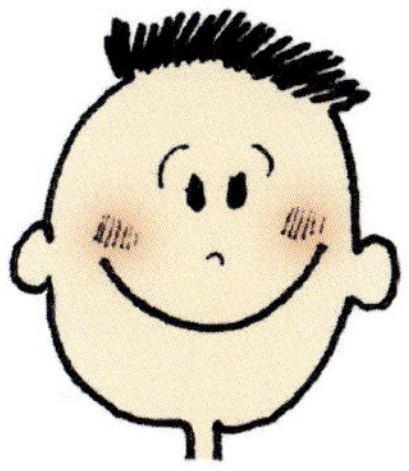 Proud
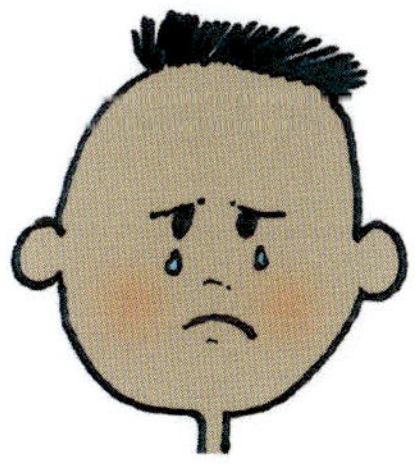 Sad	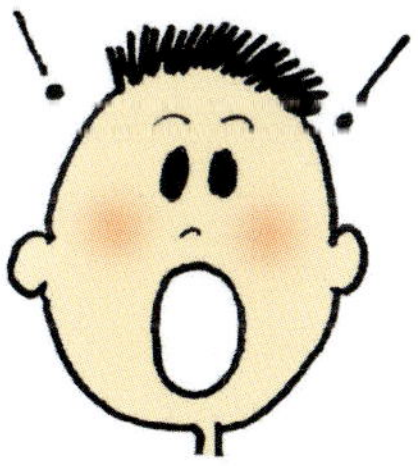 Surprised	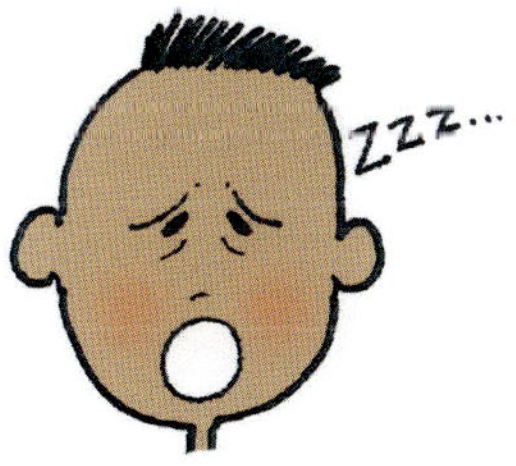 Tired
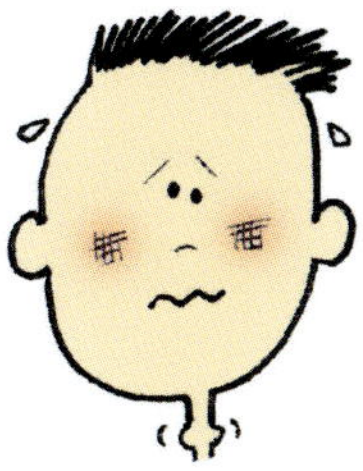 Unwell	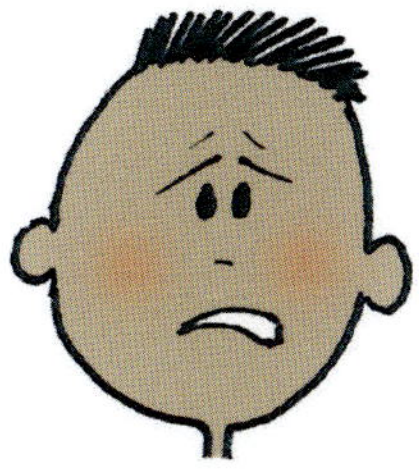 Worried	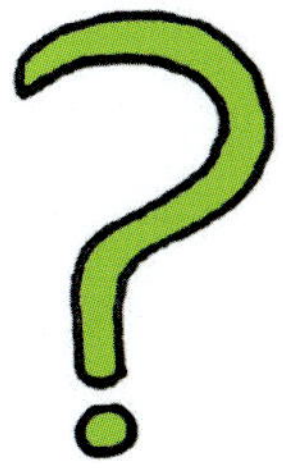 Something else

Activity 2 Who am I?

Preparation

Print out and laminate the individual cards. This activity is to help the group to get to know each other and encourage a supportive environment to share their interests and hobbies.

Instructions

- The cards are placed face down in the centre of the group.

- Each person takes a turn to pick up a card and complete the sentence.

- Continue around the group until each group member has had at least two turns.

- Choose a few to talk about as a group and for everyone to share their ideas.

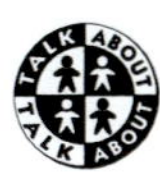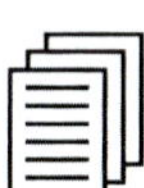

Activity 2 Who am I?

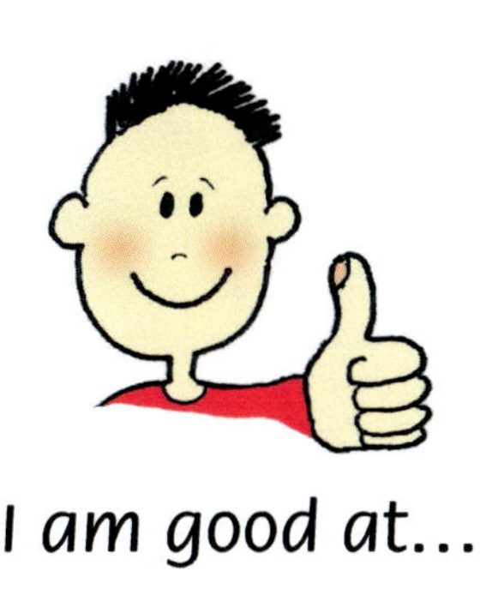

I am good at...

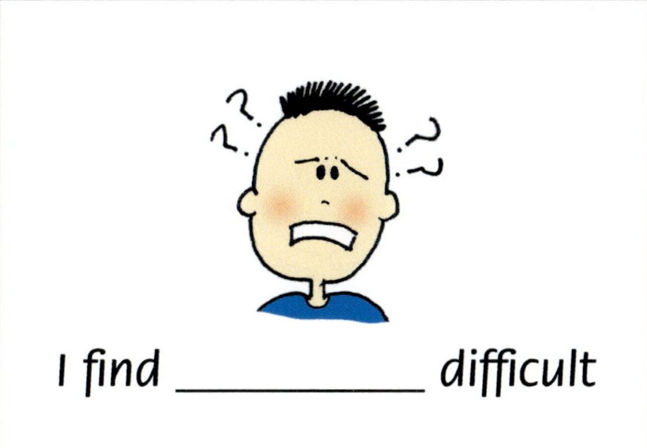

I find ___________ difficult

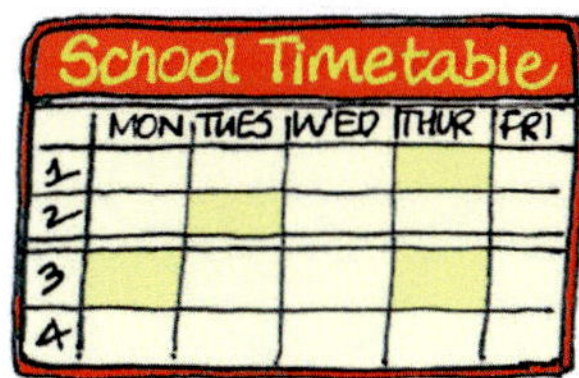

My favourite subject is...

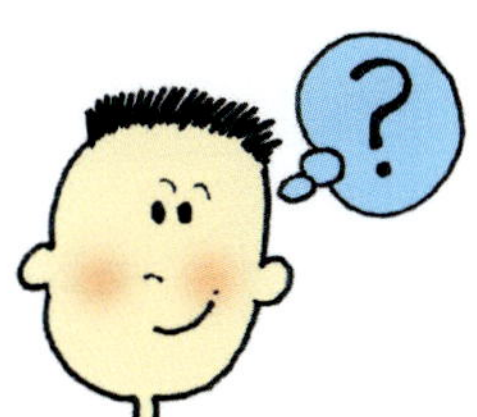

When I'm older, I want to be...

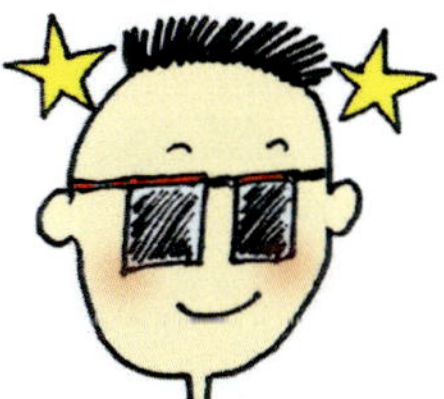

If I was to star in a TV show or film, I would most like to play...

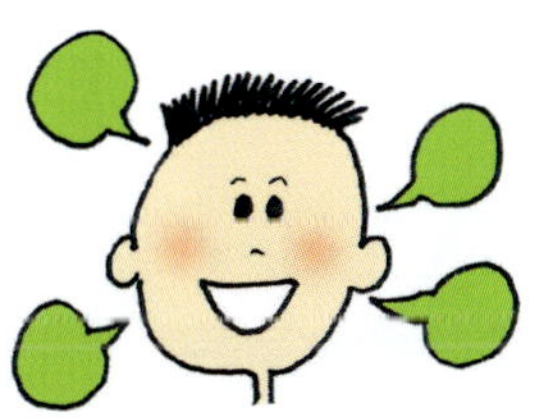

I'm interested in...

Activity 2 Who am I?

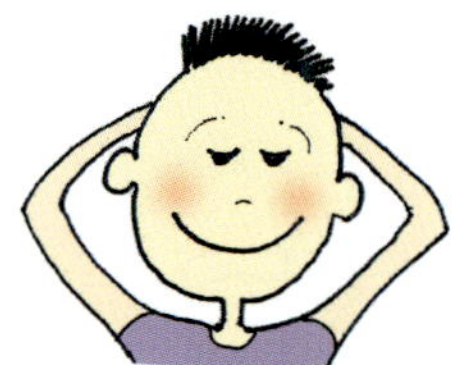

I am relaxed when…

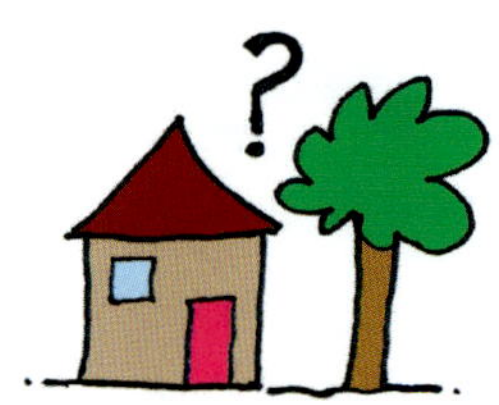

I prefer being indoors or outdoors because…

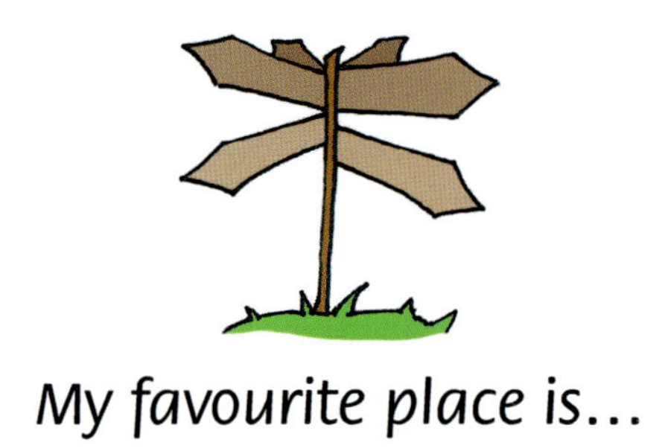

My favourite place is…

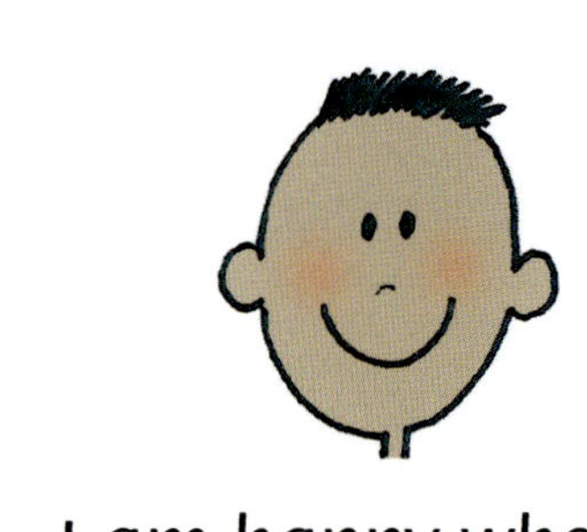

I am happy when…

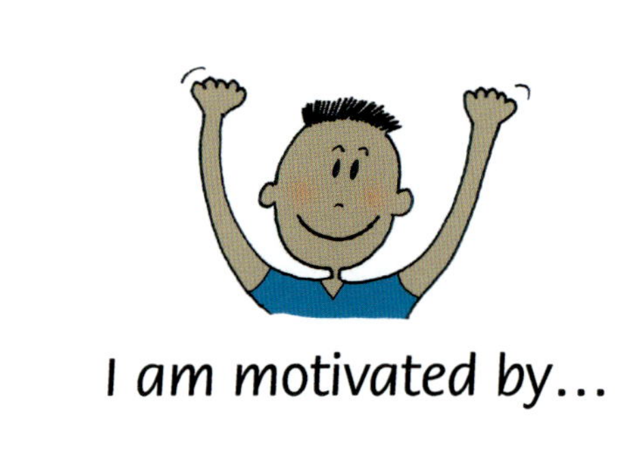

I am motivated by…

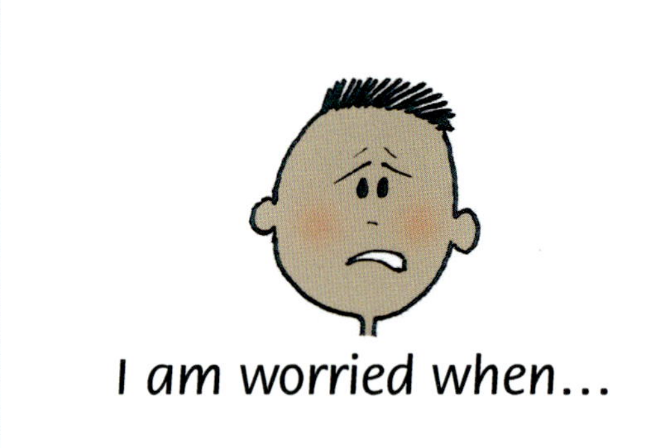

I am worried when…

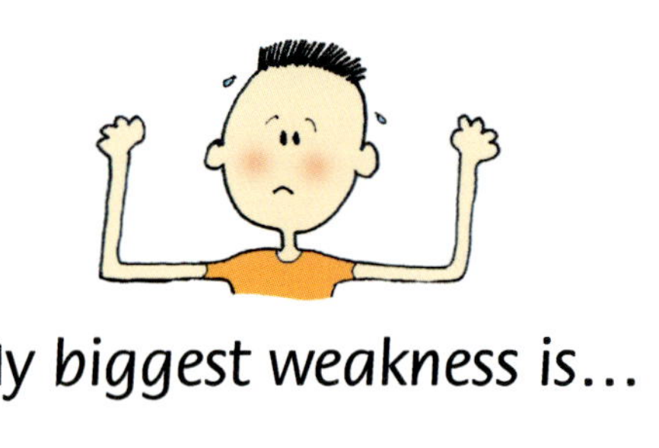

My biggest weakness is…

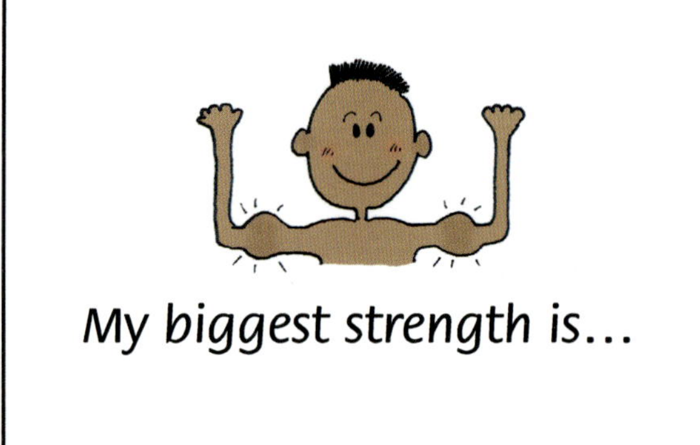

My biggest strength is…

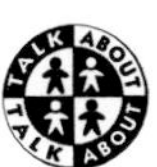
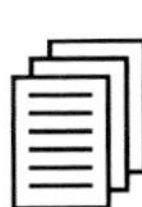

Activity 3 Where am I?

Preparation

This activity is based on the country in which your group takes place and so staff will need a rudimentary knowledge of the country's geography. If in the UK and Ireland, print out the map. If not (or if this is too broad), find a black and white outline of the country/county where the group takes place. This activity is to support group members in their self- and other awareness of their whereabouts in the world.

Instructions

- Group leaders should state that one part of the room represents a part of the country, e.g. the front of the room represents the southernmost parts of the country and the back represents the north.

- You can then explain that each member of the group is going to go around the country.

- First, ask the students to go to various important points – if in the UK and Ireland, suggest they all stand where London is, and then where Edinburgh is, and then where Cardiff, Belfast and Dublin are. Where is the Irish Sea?

- After this, ask each one where they were born and see if they know where to stand in the room. Once the students are standing there, ask them to move to where they lived when they were five, where they lived when they were ten. Finally, ask them to move to where they are now and they should all end up in the same place.

- Group members can then mark where important people in their lives live, as well as other notable locations. Some group members may have difficult relationships with their family and so it is worth remaining sensitive to this information.

- Once this is complete, ask the students to use the worksheet to mark the different locations they went to today.

Activity 3 Where am I?

Name: .... Date: ....

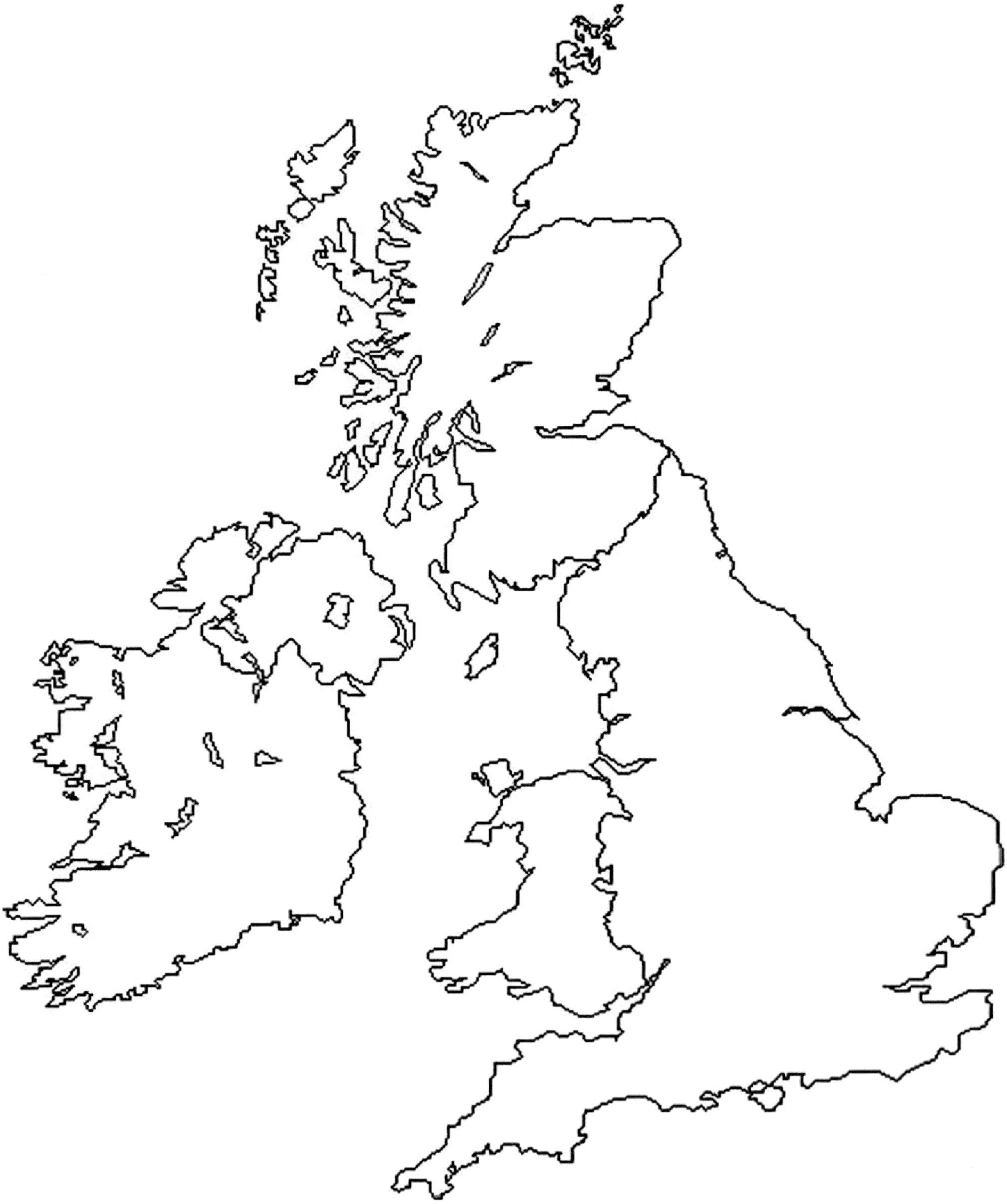

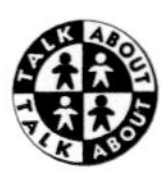
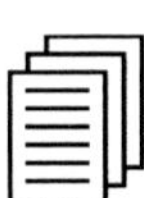

Activity 4 Useful qualities

Preparation

Photocopy, laminate and cut out the job and qualities cards. This session is to help increase group members' awareness of their own and others' qualities in relation to school, college or the workplace.

Instructions

- Introduce the concepts of 'useful' and 'not useful' by placing the title cards in the middle of the group. Explain that the group are going to discuss personality qualities that are useful to have when at work or at college/university. State that we all have lots of useful qualities that help us when we are working and that everyone has qualities that are not as useful, but that these are allowed and sometimes can be worked on.

- Introduce the jobs cards. The students can take it in turns to pick up a job card from the pile and discuss what would be a useful quality for them to have. As the group discusses each job, elicit the qualities highlighted in the next activity, e.g. hardworking, determined, clever, etc.

- These words can be written down on a flipchart/whiteboard and saved for the next session.

- Introduce the qualities cards. These can be placed in a pile in the middle of the group.

- The group members are then asked to sort the words into the two categories (although some may be disputed and can be placed in the middle).

- Take a photo of these or write these down so that they can be remembered for the next session.

Activity 4 Useful qualities

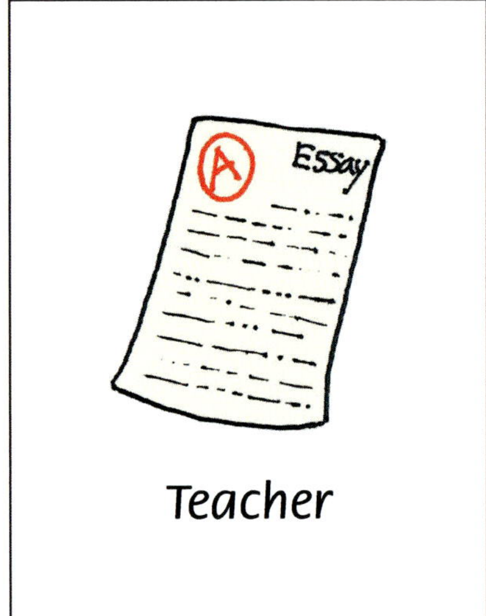

Teacher

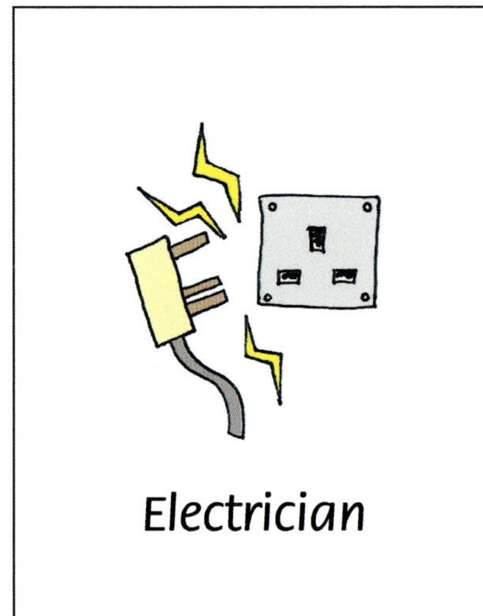

Electrician

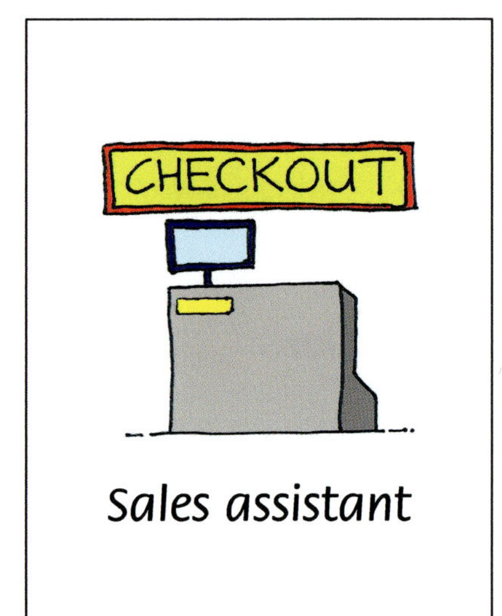

Sales assistant

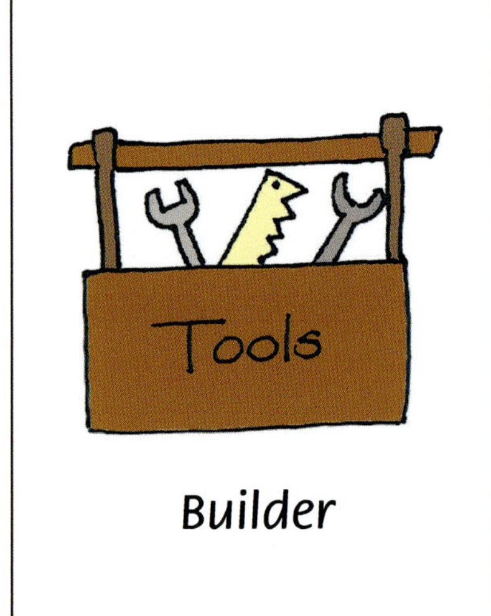

Builder

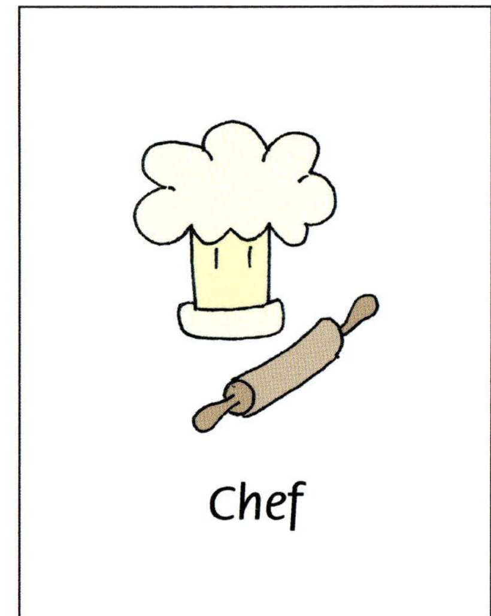

Chef

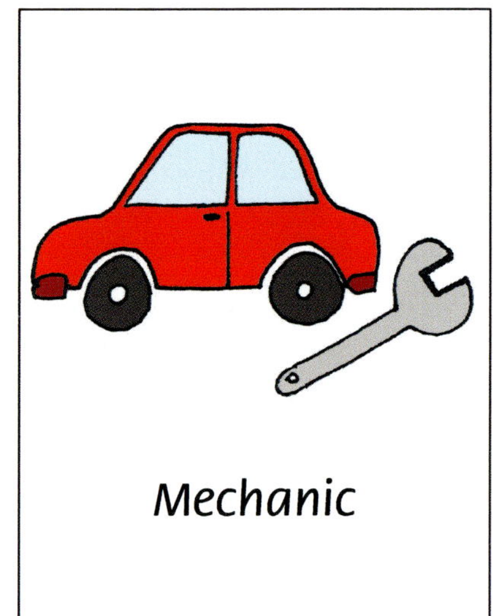

Mechanic

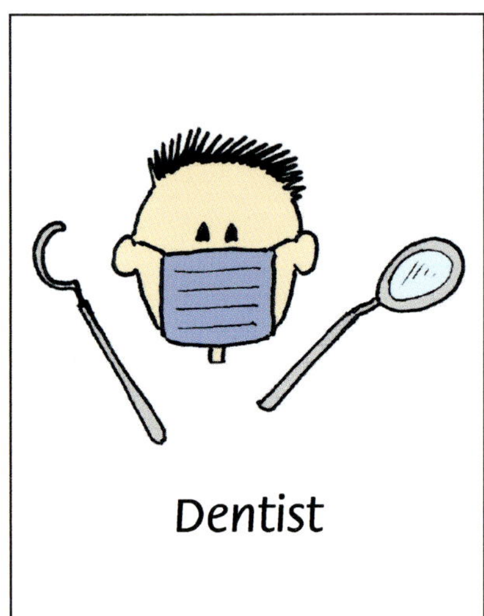

Dentist

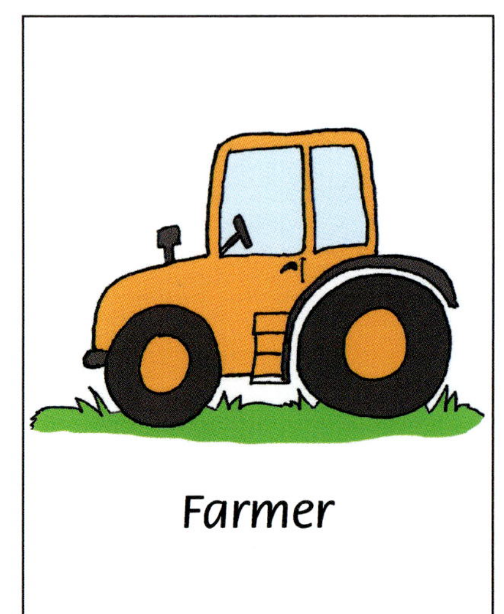

Farmer

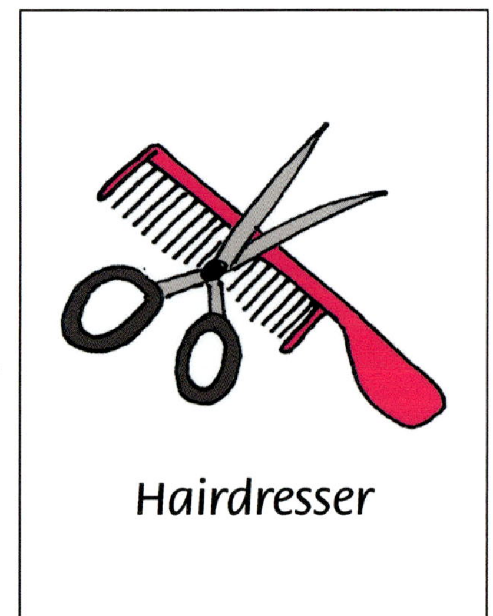

Hairdresser

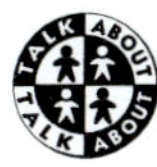
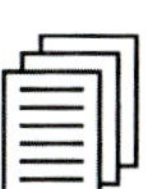

Activity 4 Useful qualities

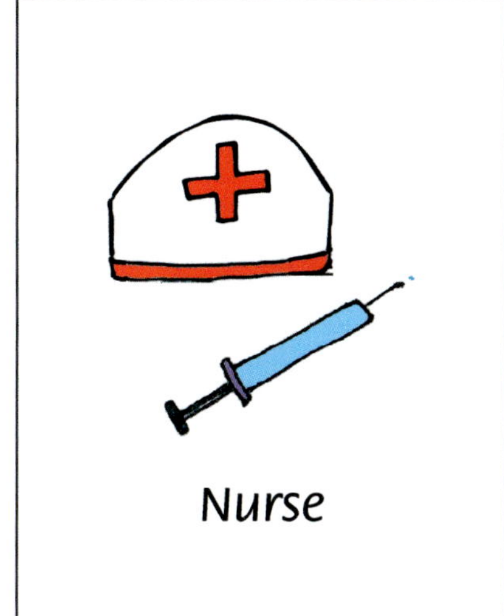

Nurse

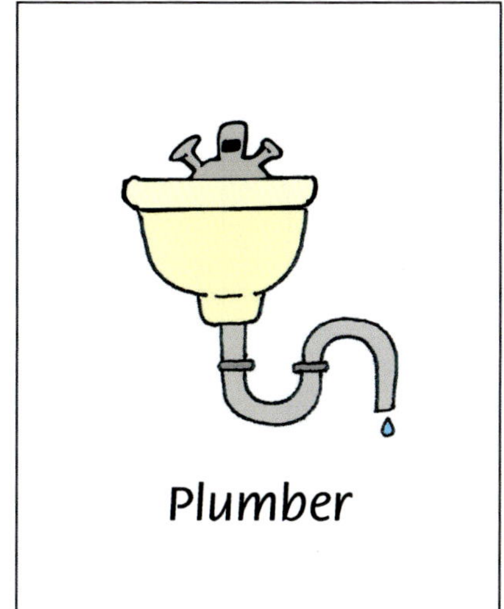

Plumber

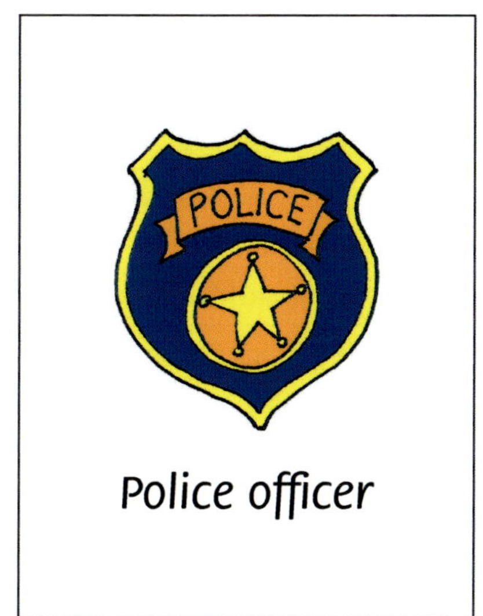

Police officer

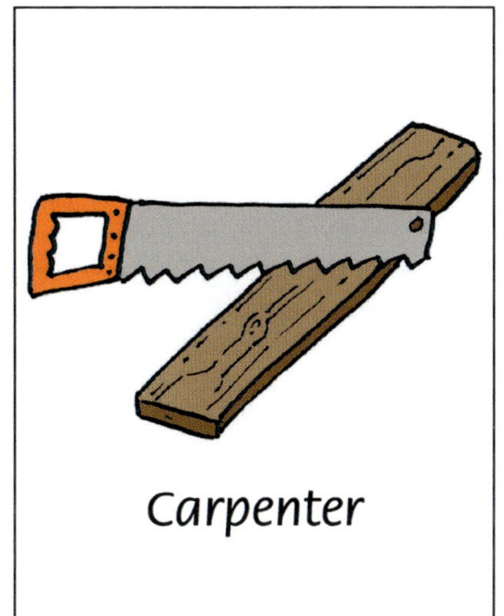

Carpenter

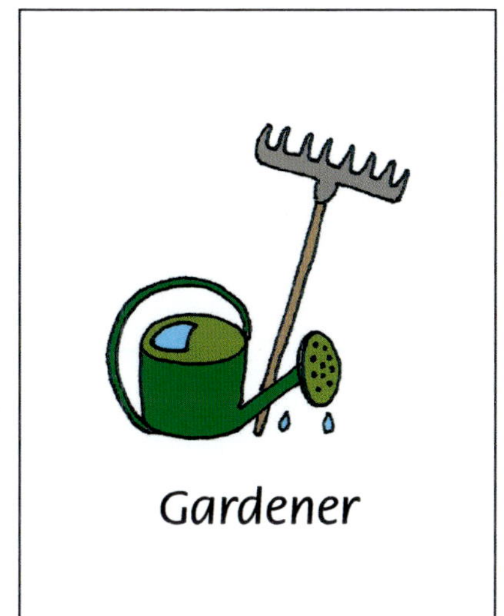

Gardener

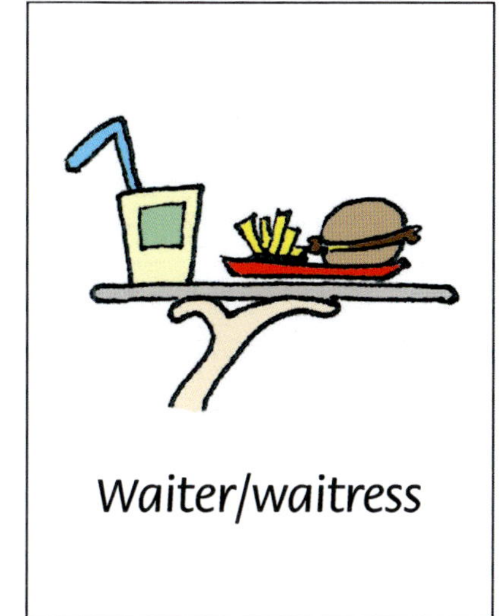

Waiter/waitress

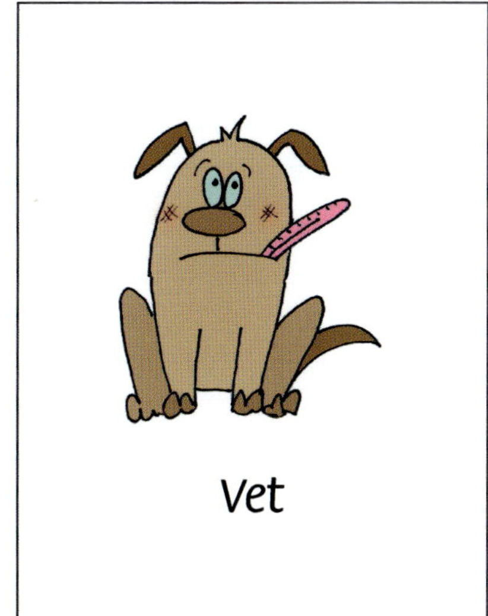

Vet

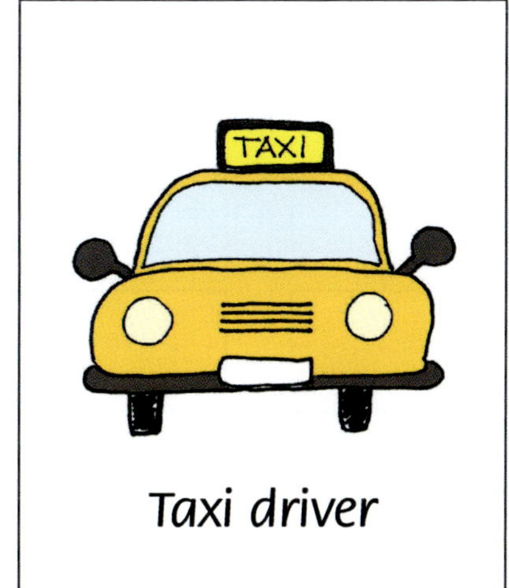

Taxi driver

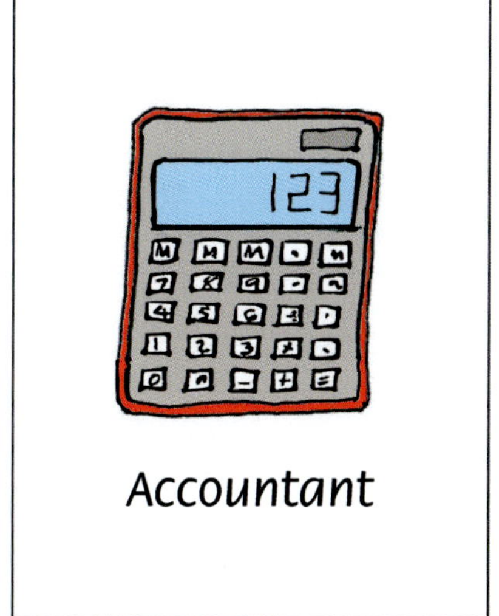

Accountant

Activity 4 Useful qualities

Qualities that are useful	Qualities that aren't useful
Honest	Opinionated
Hardworking	Organised
Flexible	Enthusiastic
Determined	Clever
Friendly	Silly
Lazy	Joker
Open minded	Creative
Confident	Impatient
Easy going	Sensitive
Quiet	Helpful
Talkative	Serious
Unfriendly	Unfocused
Good listener	Nervous
Bossy	Responsible

Activity 5 My qualities

Preparation

Photocopy the worksheet. Use the qualities cards from Activity 4.

Instructions

- Provide the group members with a worksheet and ask them to choose which qualities from the previous session would best describe them. They can use the cards as prompts or come up with original ones.

- It would then be useful for each group member to think of one quality that they could work on.

- Group members might like to share their worksheet with someone they trust. Do the others agree with the words they circled?

Activity 5 My qualities

Name: .... Date: ....

....

....

....

My qualities

....

....

....

One quality that isn't useful that I think I could work on is:

....

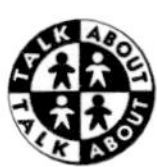

Activity 6 What do I like to do?

Preparation

Photocopy the worksheet. Use the qualities cards from Activity 4 and photocopy, laminate and cut out the skills cards in this activity.

Instructions

- Start a discussion between group members around what hobbies or interests they have at home or at school. Discuss what they like to do and what motivates them.

- Give the worksheets out and ask the group members to write their favourite hobby on the top of the worksheet (if they can't choose, they can use more than one worksheet).

- Group members should look at the skills cards. What skills do they need to carry out this task? For example, if their favourite activity is playing video games, they might be good at using a computer and doing lots of different things all at once, as well as independently doing an activity. If they like playing football, they might be good at working in a team and have good physical skills. The group members can then either write these in the boxes on the worksheet or cut and stick the options from the individual cards.

- After this, group members should identify the qualities that they have which are useful in relation to this hobby. For example, if they like going shopping they might be enthusiastic, open minded and creative. If they like English lessons, they might be clever, talkative and hardworking. The group members can then either write these in the boxes on the worksheet or cut and stick the options from the individual cards.

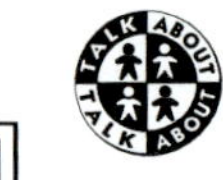

Activity 6 What do I like to do?

Name: .... Date: ....

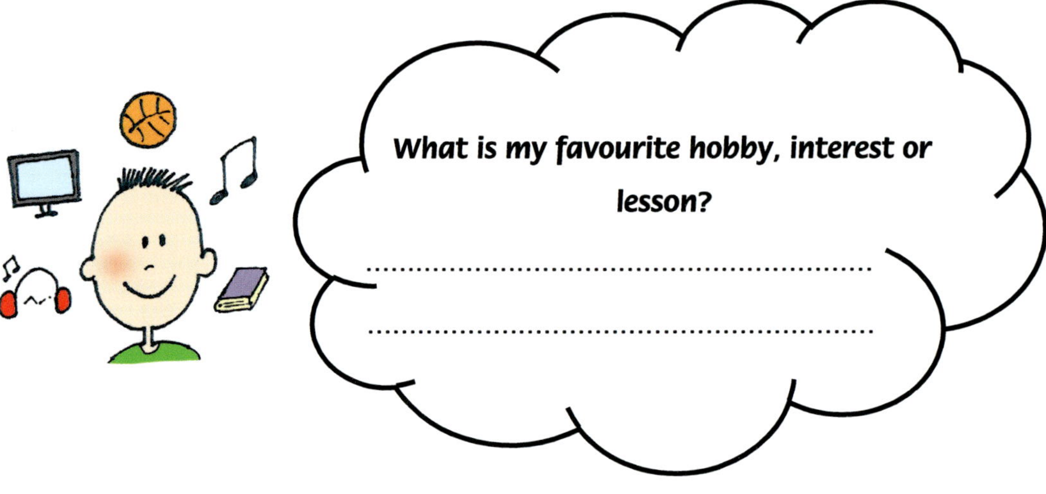

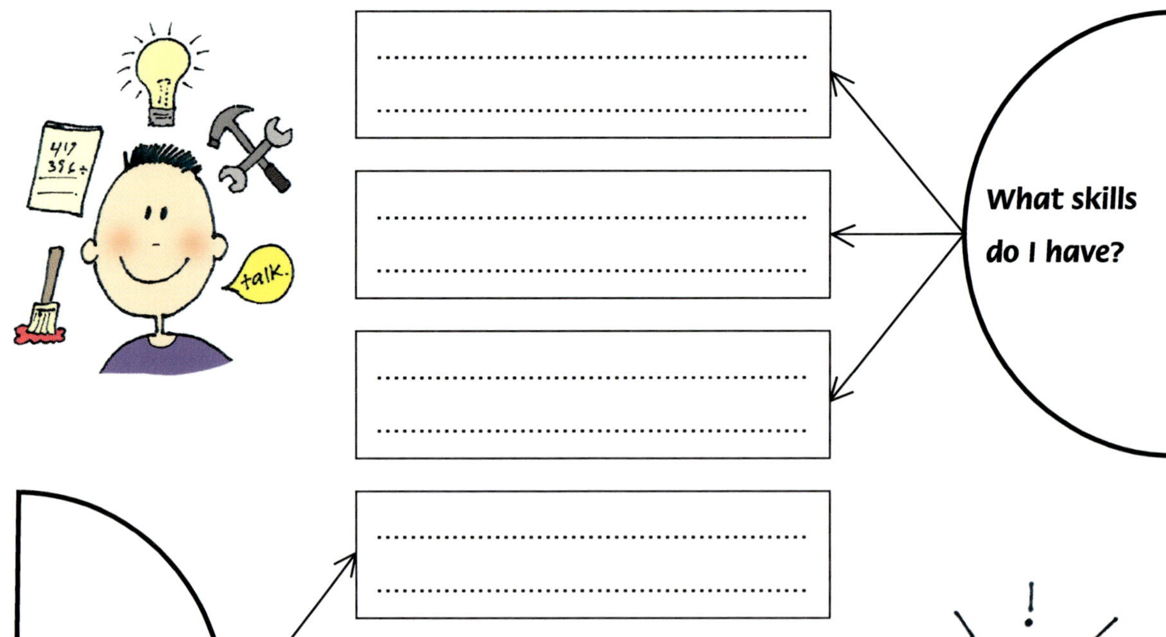

Activity 6 What do I like to do?

Listening to instructions	Speaking to people
Writing and spelling	Reading
Working with other people	Solving a problem in different ways
Thinking about how to do lots of different things at once	Using a computer, tablet or phone
Thinking about how to do something new or differently	Doing maths
Using physical skills, e.g. hand -eye coordination or stamina	Taking the initiative or making decisions
Being independent	Changing or adapting your behaviour when you need to
Planning how to do something	Listening to other people
Attempting a task repeatedly until successful	Other...

Activity 7 Advertise me

Preparation

Photocopy the worksheet or ask the group members to create their own advert on plain/ coloured paper. If appropriate, and if the group members would like to, use a video camera or mobile phone to record their advert.

Instructions

- Explain to the group that they will be creating an advert for themselves, explaining all the good qualities about them and what they like doing. They can use the worksheet from Activity 6 as a prompt if they can't remember. They may like to complete their own separate poster, but they should still include the same information.

- After this, the group members can give feedback to the rest of the group. One other option includes recording the group members doing short individual adverts, around 30 seconds long, on a video camera/mobile phone. This would involve reading out their description to advertise their qualities and skills, and then watching it back with the group.

- Keep these posters for activities in later topics.

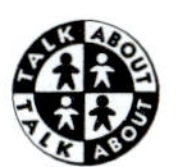
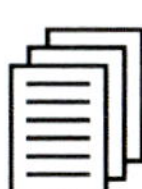

Activity 7 Advertise me

Name: ....

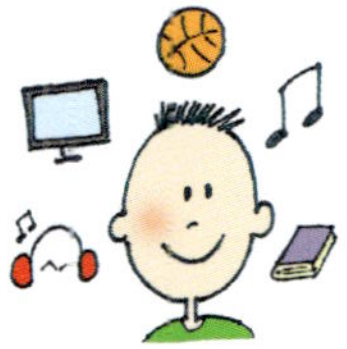

Date: ....

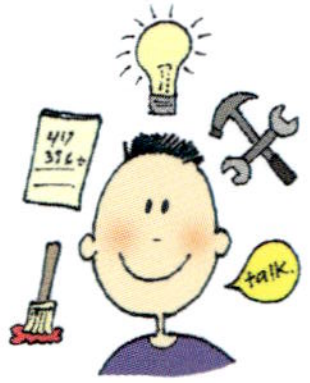

This is me ....

My skills

My interests

My qualities

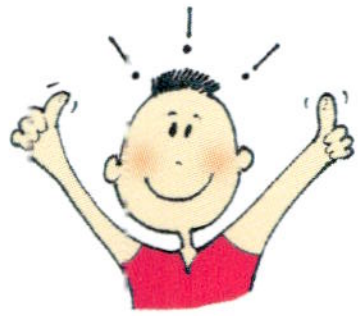

One thing I could work on

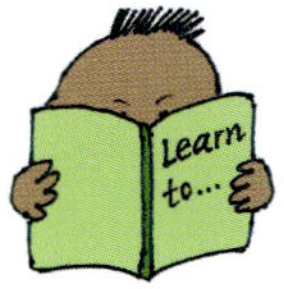

Topic 2 – Which route do I take?

Objectives

To understand the difference between the different routes available when the group members leave school or college.

To explore different employment choices and identify interesting and realistic jobs that the group members could do based on their interests, skills and qualities.

To identify what skills or qualifications the group members will need to achieve their chosen career choice.

Timing

This topic will take up to eight sessions to complete.

Activity	Description
Help me choose! (Activity 8)	The group leaders read out a character's scenario and the group members decide which route would be the best choice for the character.
Guess who I am (Activity 9)	Each group member takes it in turns to read out a description of a job and the group members guess what it is.
Twenty questions (Activity 10)	The group members ask questions to one group member to figure out what occupation they are.
Naming jobs (Activity 11)	The group members name as many jobs as they can think of and pick three that they think they'd like to try.
Choosing a job (Activity 12)	Each group member thinks about how their interests, skills and qualities will help them do their chosen jobs.
How do we get there? (Activity 13)	The group members look at a selection of careers and decide which route they need to go down to achieve this.
Which route can I take? (Activity 14)	The group members fill in individual worksheets based on the different routes, weighing up the pros and cons of each route.
Next steps (Activity 15)	Each group member thinks about one of the jobs they chose and fills in a worksheet to show what their next steps would be to achieve this.

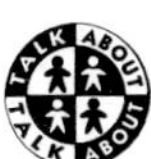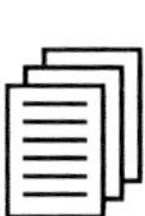

Activity 8 Help me choose!

Preparation

Photocopy the scenario cards or read them from the book. Either print out and laminate one copy of the options boxes or print out and laminate a copy of the option boxes for each group member.

Instructions

- Place the options boxes in the middle of the group or provide each member of the group with a copy of all six options.

- The group leaders read through each individual scenario.

- The group leaders can then either read out all the individual options printed below the scenario and ask the students to choose which route they could take; or the students can look at the options in the middle of the group and decide together what the person could do, elaborating on each point (e.g. What are they going to study at university? What job will they look at?); or the students can use their cards to vote for what they think the person should do in the scenario. They can do this by choosing the card in secret and putting all the cards in the middle. The group leaders then encourage the group members to discuss what decisions they have made and why they think this is the correct decision.

- Group members can choose more than one option if they feel it is appropriate or they are not sure.

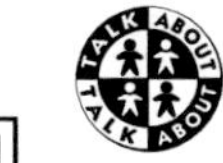

Activity 8 Help me choose!

Lizzie is in her last term at school. She hates school because she has been bullied by her classmates. She tries hard in her lessons but struggles to get good grades. When she leaves, she hopes to get two GCSEs. Lizzie is quiet and shy but is very friendly and loves animals. What do you think Lizzie could try?

A) Go to college and do A-levels to try and do Veterinary Medicine at university

B) Go to the pet shop and see if there are any vacancies for work

C) Look into apprenticeships at the local vets practice

D) Approach a local farmer to ask about work experience

E) Go to the job centre to claim unemployment benefit

Ismael is going into his final year of A-levels at his sixth form college. He has just had his AS results, consisting of an A, B and C in English, Psychology and Biology. When Ismael finishes college he hopes to have the same grades. He likes to have a laugh and enjoys reading. Where do you think Ismael should go?

A) Go to the job centre to claim unemployment benefit

B) Apply to university to do an English course

C) Go on a foundation course at college before he goes to university

D) Apply for a job at a local restaurant to work as a chef

E) Volunteer at a local charity to get some work experience

Activity 8 Help me choose!

Mo is in his last year at school. He likes going to school to see his friends but is quite naughty and doesn't listen all the time in his lessons, especially Maths and English, which are difficult for him. His favourite lessons are woodwork and cooking and he works better when he is able to get 'hands on'. What should Mo do at the end of the year?

A) Go to the job centre to claim unemployment benefit

B) Go to college to do a foundation course in a practical subject, such as brick-laying or mechanics

C) Go to a local carpentry company and volunteer for work experience

D) Talk to the careers advisor at school and see if there are any possibilities of apprenticeships in the area

E) Apply to his sixth form college to do academic subjects

Katie has nearly finished her A-levels and has a place to go to university in September to study Psychology. She doesn't like going to school and was pressured into going to university because all her friends are going. Katie would like to earn money to go travelling instead. What should Katie do?

A) Carry on with her course and see if she likes it in September

B) Apply to carry out a foundation course at a college

C) Drop from her course and claim benefits from the job centre

D) Give CVs to local companies in the town to see if she can get a job

E) See if she can volunteer at a local charity

Activity 8 Help me choose!

Summer is about to finish her GCSEs. Summer hates school because she finds it difficult to listen and doesn't have many friends. She doesn't know what she would like to do or what she is good at and will probably not have any GCSEs when she finishes. What could she do to help herself?

A) Pass CVs out among local businesses to apply for jobs

B) Volunteer at local charities to see if she likes taking part in the community

C) Talk to her school careers advisor to discuss her future

D) Finish school and see if she can find work at the job centre

E) Apply to a local college to do an entry level or foundation course

Shameera has finished her A-levels and passed all of them. She is very musically talented and can play lots of different instruments. She currently sings in a popular local band. What should Shameera do?

A) Continue to just play in the band around her local area

B) Apply to a music course at university to see if she can get better and meet new band mates

C) Apply to work at local music shops

D) Volunteer at local charities to play music in the community

E) Leave the band and stay at home

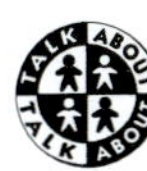
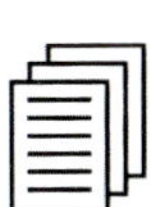

Activity 8 Help me choose!

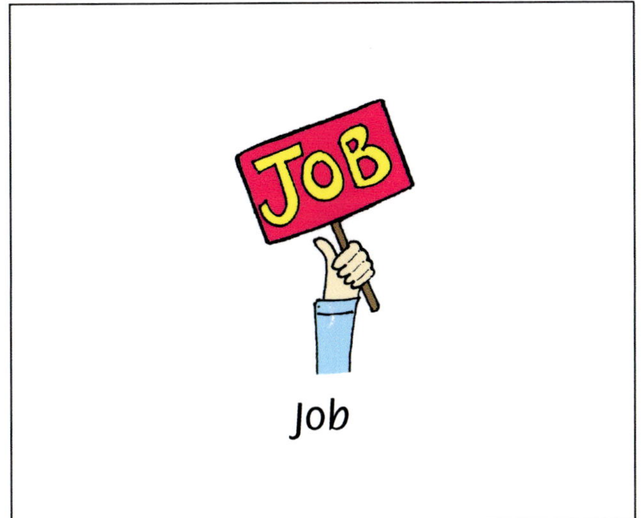

Job

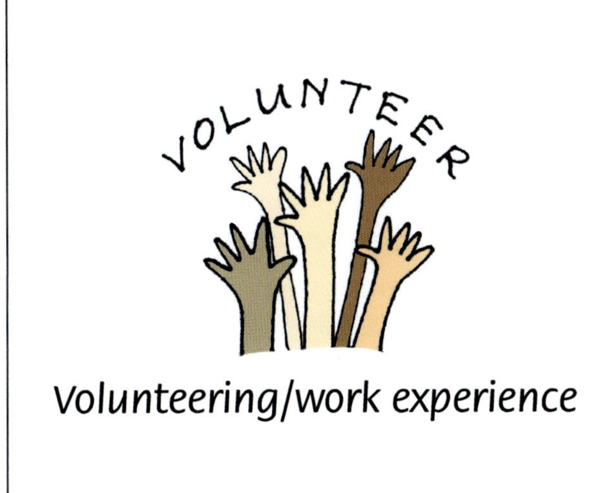

Volunteering/work experience

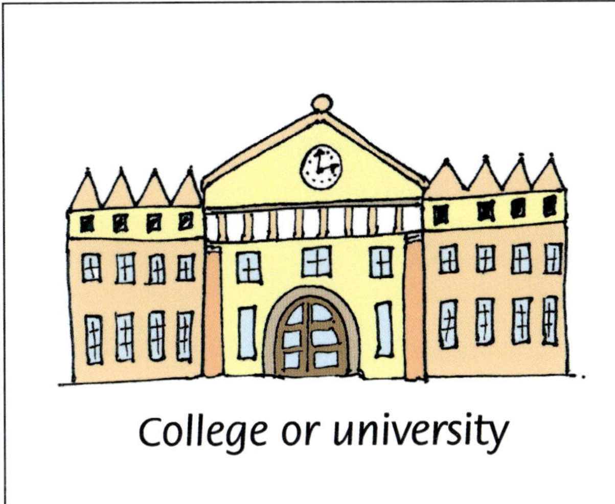

College or university

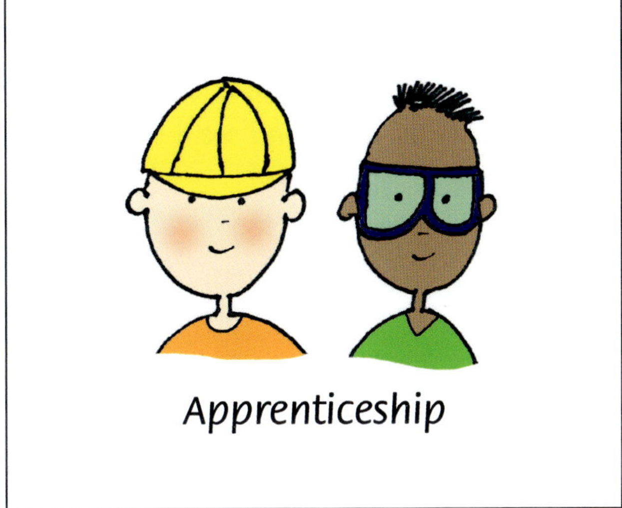

Apprenticeship

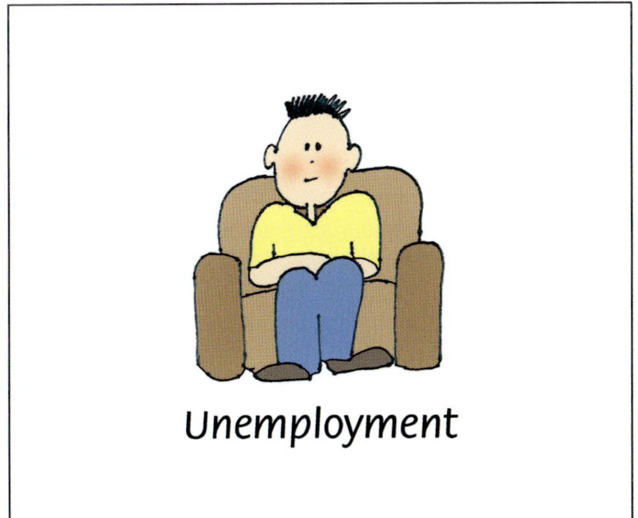

Unemployment

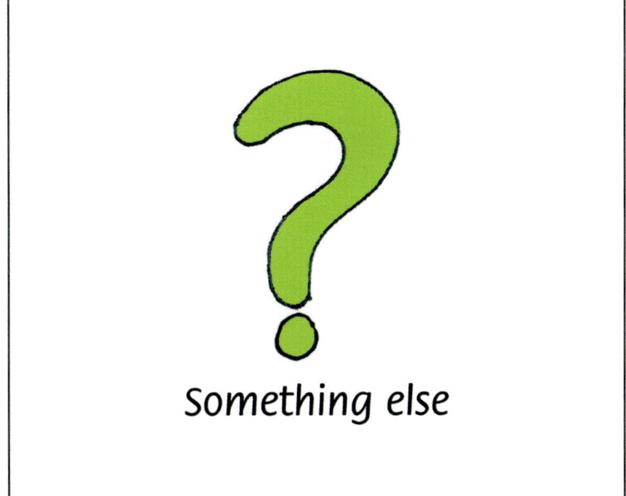

Something else

Activity 9 Guess who I am?

Preparation

Photocopy and laminate the cards.

Instructions

- Each group member takes a turn to pick a card. On their turn, they read out one clue at a time from the card. After they have read out each clue, each member of the group takes a turn to guess what they might be.

- The group members only get one guess per clue, so if they use it too quickly, they can't guess again until the next clue!

- Continue until the pile of cards runs out.

- To expand this activity, see if each group member can come up with their own profession and six ways to describe it. Once they have done this, each group member takes a turn to read out their clues and see if the other group members can guess what they are.

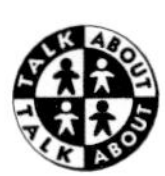

Activity 9 Guess who I am?

---

1. I go to houses or places of work to speak to lots of different people.
2. I am very observant and careful in certain situations.
3. I drive cars, vans and motorcycles.
4. I interview people.
5. I go to court and give evidence.
6. I carry handcuffs to arrest people.
7. I am a police officer.

---

1. I advise people on how they can look good.
2. I use lots of equipment to help people look how they want.
3. I make appointments in person and over the phone.
4. I work with dyes and chemicals.
5. I use a mirror, comb, brush and hairdryer.
6. I wash and cut hair.
7. I am a hairdresser.

---

1. People must be able to trust me.
2. I monitor people 24 hours a day.
3. I must respond quickly to emergencies.
4. I write healthcare plans for patients.
5. I prepare people for operations, treat wounds and give injections.
6. I work in hospitals or the community.
7. I am a nurse.

---

1. I work very long days.
2. I work outside all year round and deal with all weathers.
3. I do basic maintenance on vehicles and fences, gates or walls.
4. I might work with animals.
5. I might have to plant and harvest crops.
6. I drive a tractor.
7. I am a farmer.

---

1. I work in homes and other buildings.
2. I make sure buildings are safe.
3. I use hand tools and power tools.
4. I make sure people don't use dangerous equipment.
5. I repair broken appliances.
6. I test, maintain and connect electrical wiring.
7. I am an electrician.

---

1. I can work outdoors and indoors.
2. I operate machinery.
3. I work as part of a team.
4. Sometimes I work through bad weather.
5. I might do maintenance jobs, make safer roads or create houses.
6. I have to wear protective equipment, like a hard hat.
7. I am a builder.

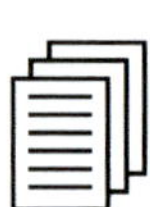
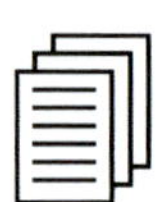

Activity 9 Guess who I am?

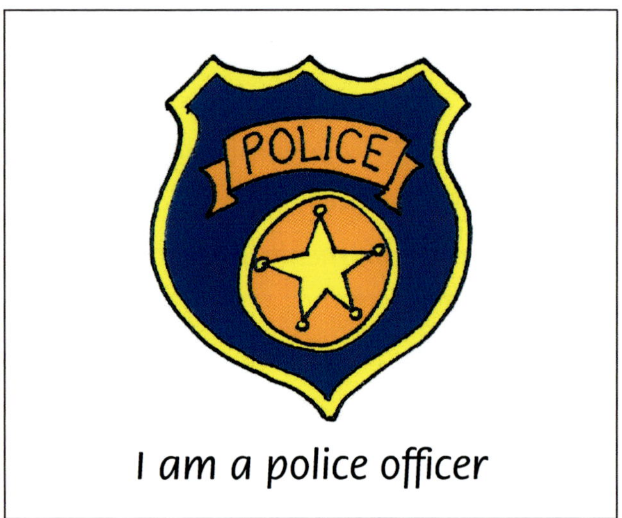

I am a police officer

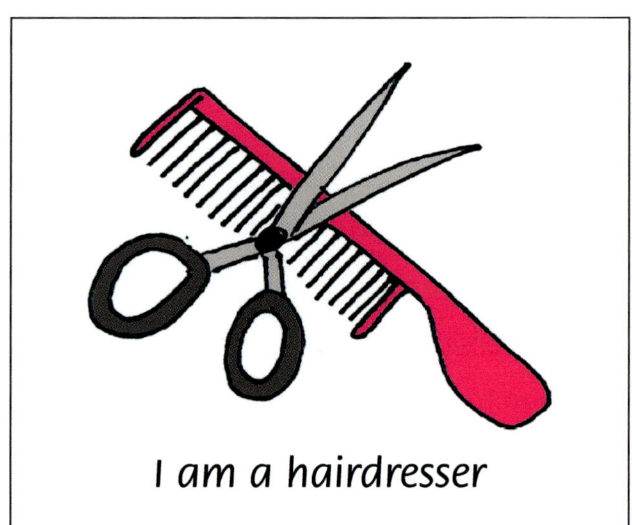

I am a hairdresser

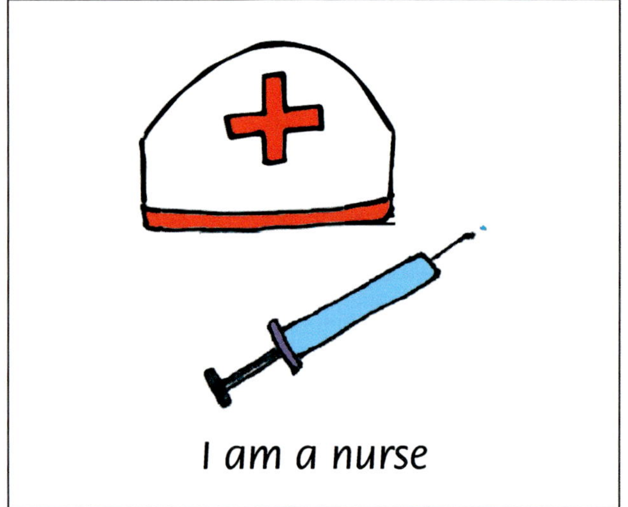

I am a nurse

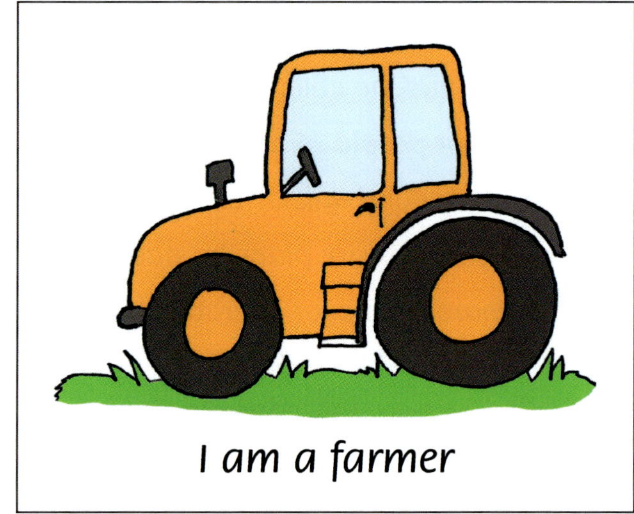

I am a farmer

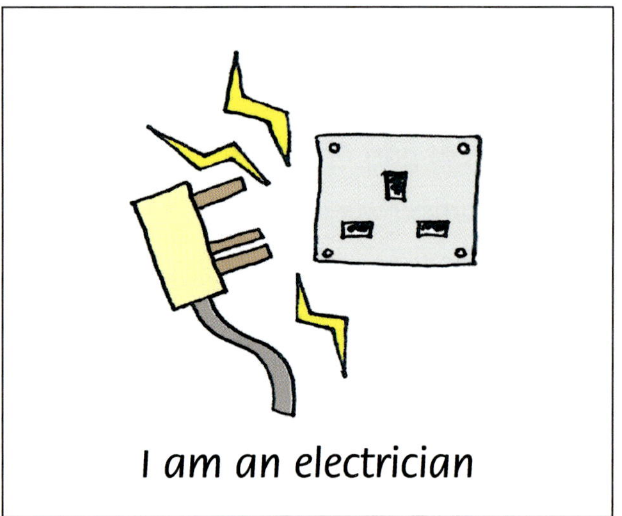

I am an electrician

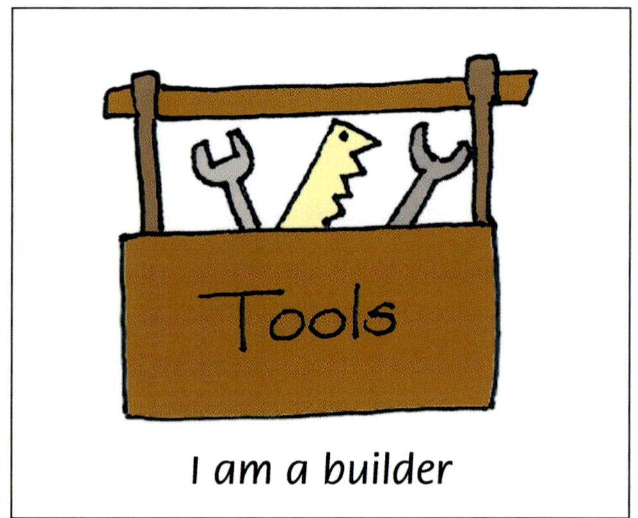

I am a builder

Activity 10 Twenty questions

Preparation

Print, laminate and cut out the individual occupation cards (these are worth keeping as you can reuse them in Activity 13). Print out a word map for each student or make it A3 so that everyone can see it.

Instructions

- Each group member takes a turn to pick a card. Once they have taken a card, the other group members will take it in turns to ask them questions to find out what profession is on their card.

- To do this, either the group can come up with their own questions or use the question map as prompts for questions. The questions can only be 'yes' or 'no' questions and that is the only way the group member whose turn it is can answer.

- The students have 20 questions to find out what the answer is, although, if appropriate, carry on until they have figured out the answer. To make it slightly easier, the group member can answer more open questions instead of just 'yes' or 'no' questions.

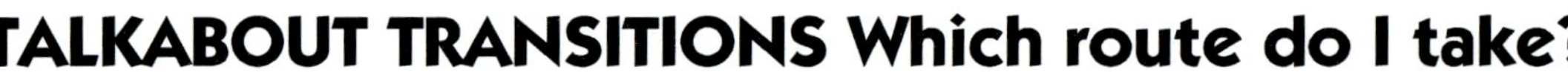
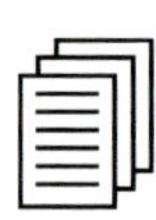

Activity 10 Twenty questions

Teacher 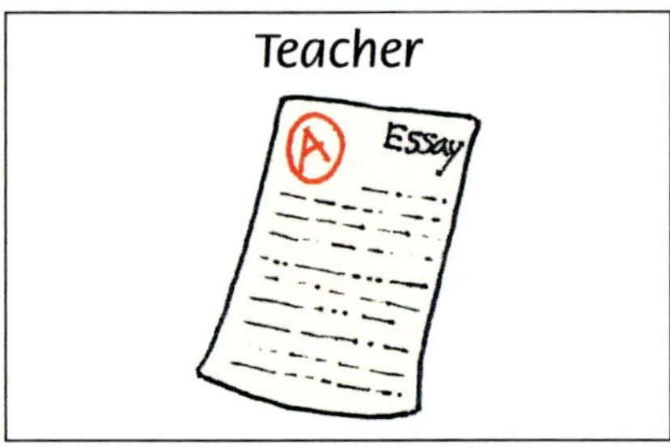	Electrician 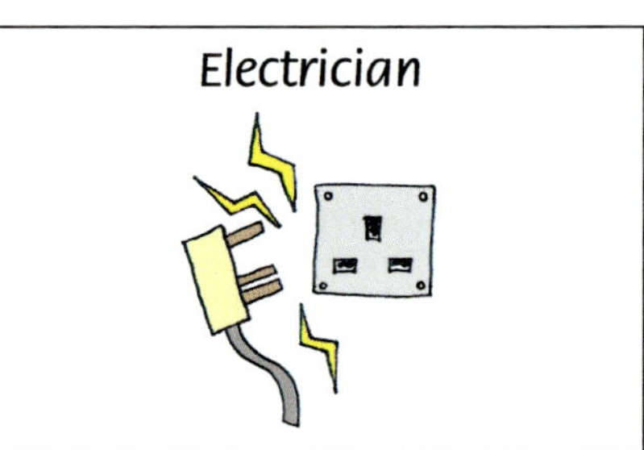	Sales assistant 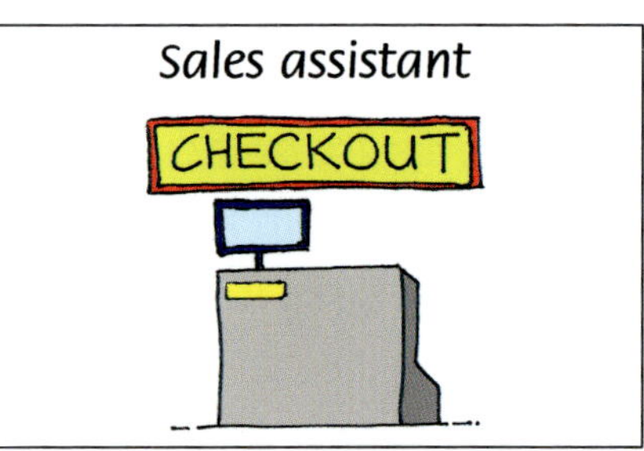
Builder 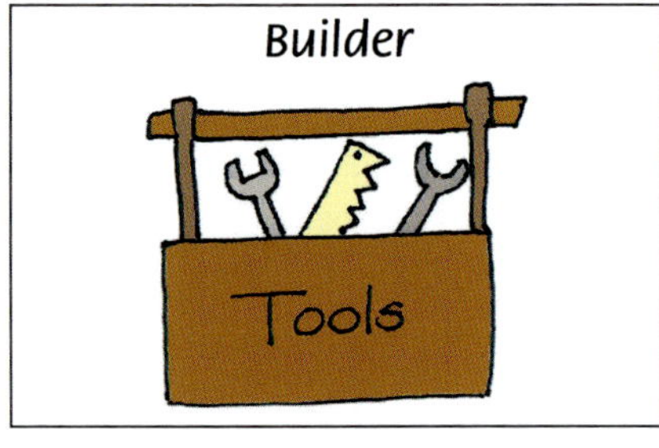	Chef 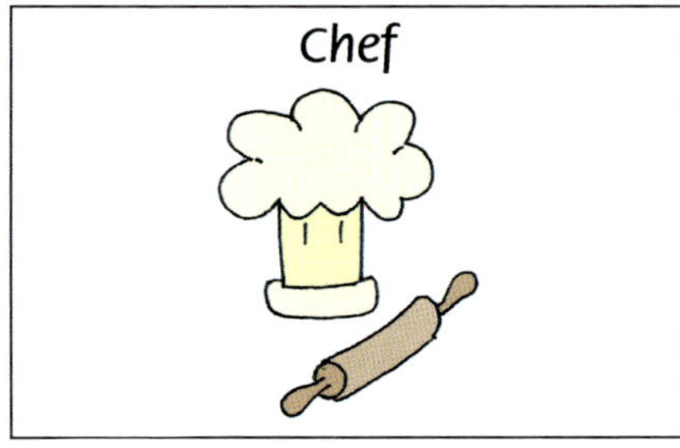	Mechanic 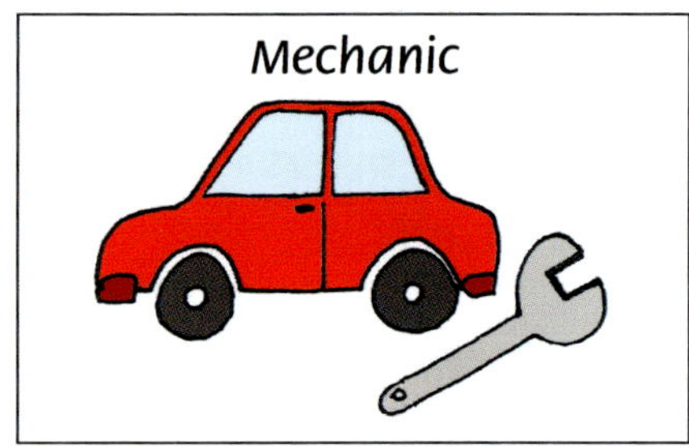
Dentist 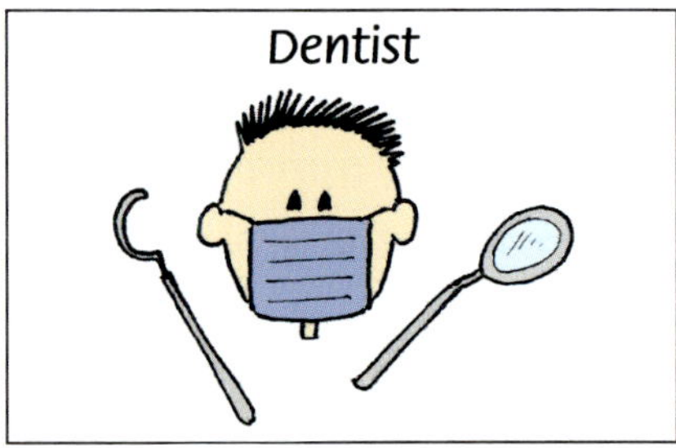	Farmer 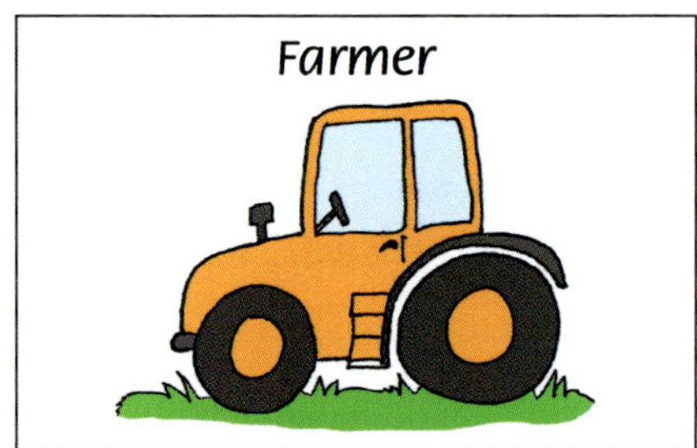	Hairdresser 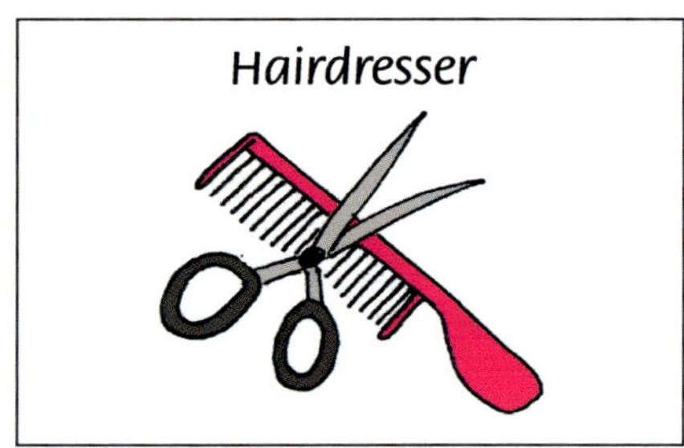
Nurse 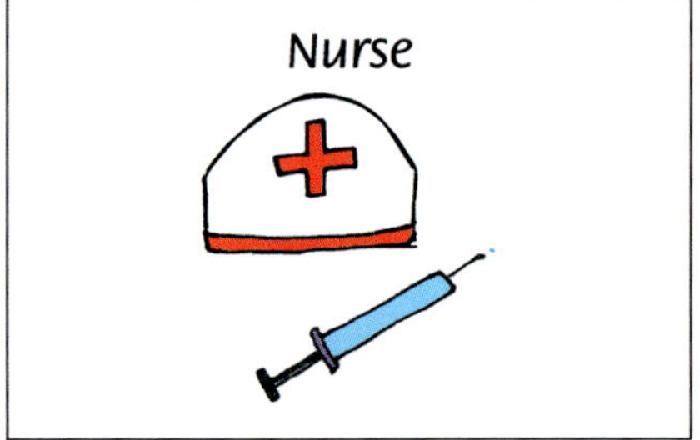	Plumber 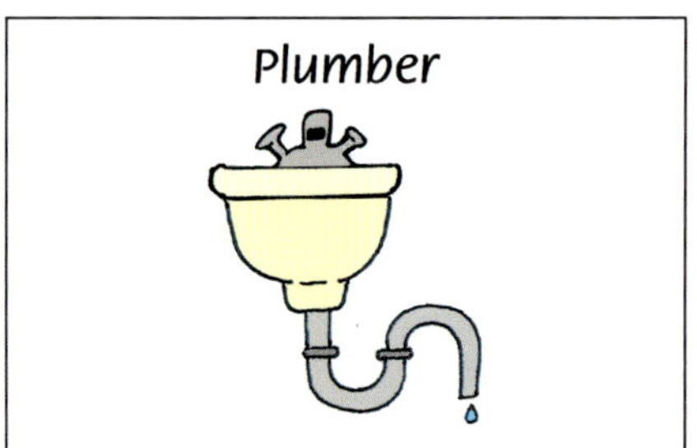	Police officer 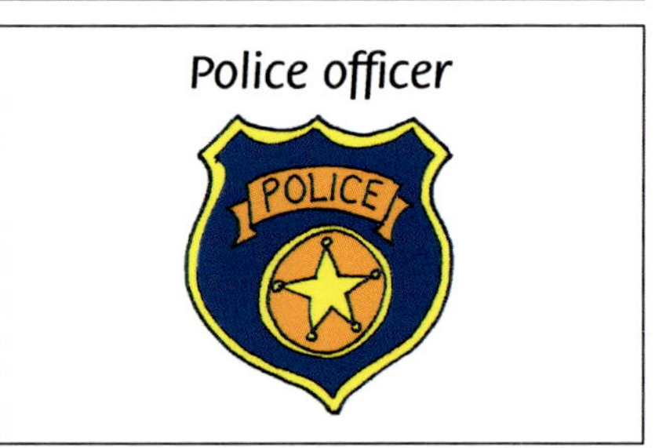
Carpenter 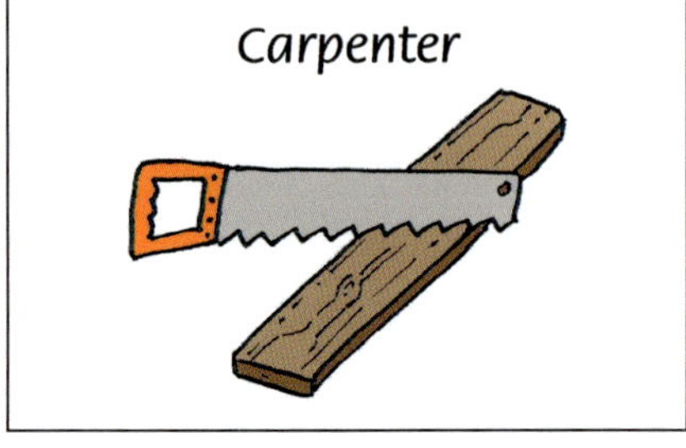	Gardener 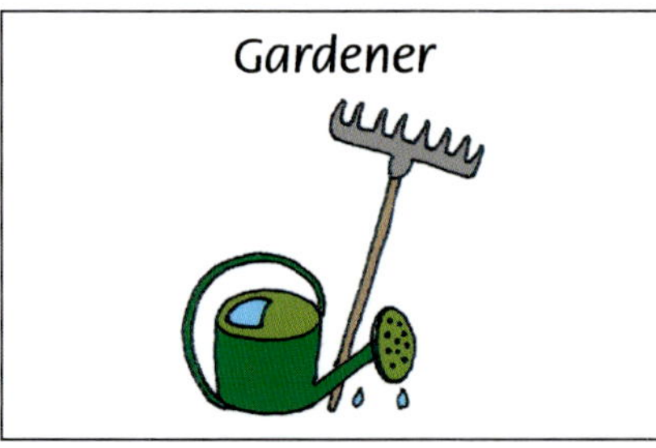	Waiter/waitress 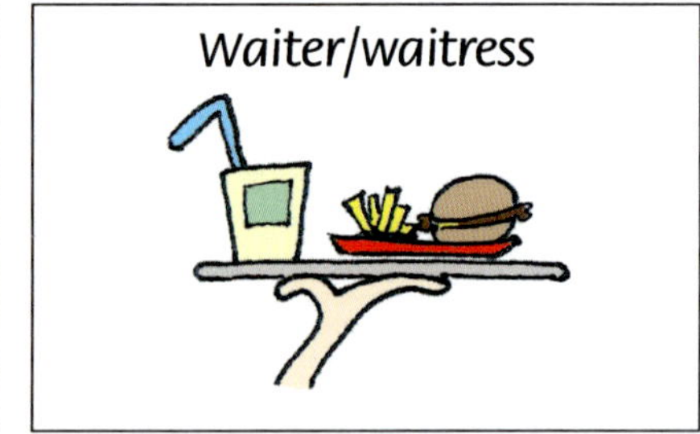
Vet 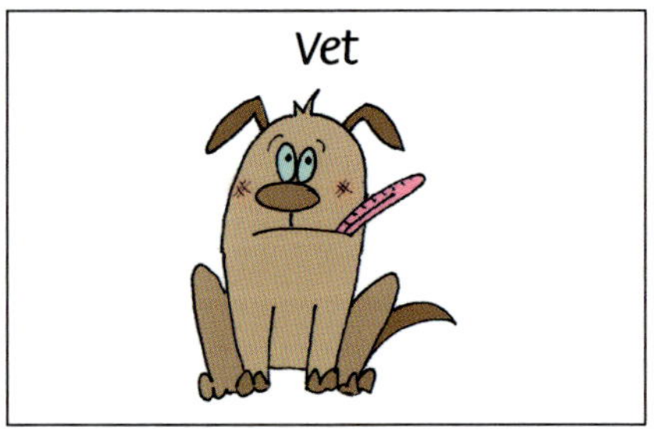	Taxi driver 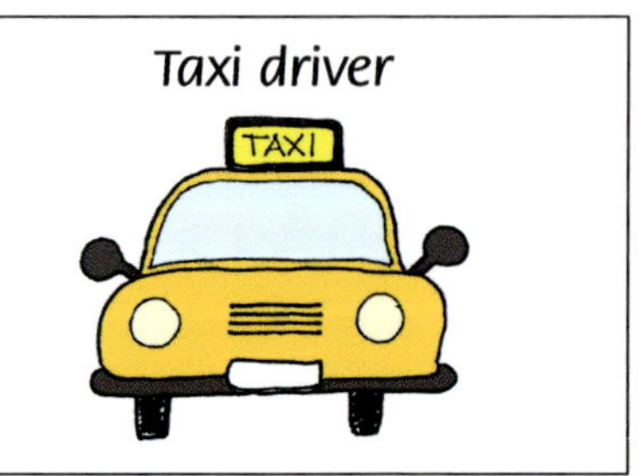	Accountant 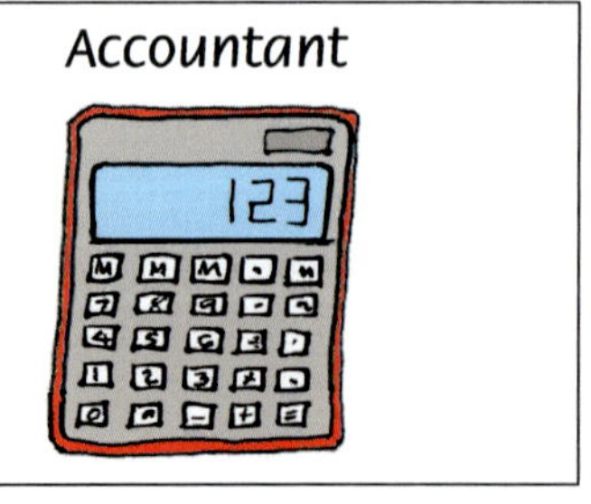

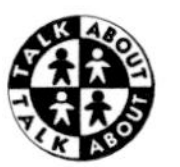
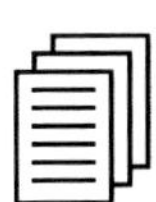

Activity 10 Twenty questions

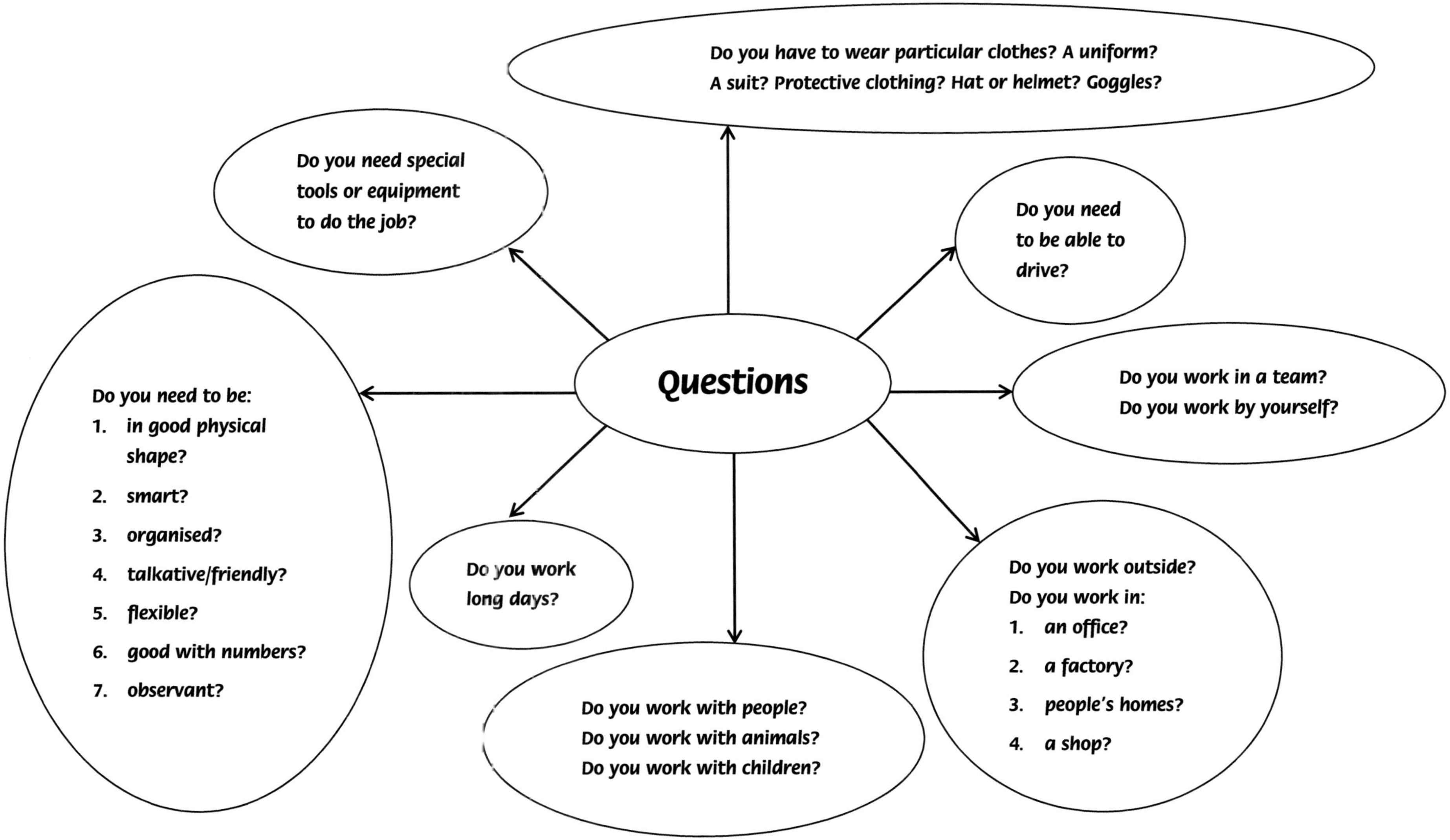

Questions

Do you have to wear particular clothes? A uniform? A suit? Protective clothing? Hat or helmet? Goggles?

Do you need to be able to drive?

Do you work in a team? Do you work by yourself?

Do you work outside?
Do you work in:
1. an office?
2. a factory?
3. people's homes?
4. a shop?

Do you work with people?
Do you work with animals?
Do you work with children?

Do you work long days?

Do you need special tools or equipment to do the job?

Do you need to be:
1. in good physical shape?
2. smart?
3. organised?
4. talkative/friendly?
5. flexible?
6. good with numbers?
7. observant?

Activity 11 Jobs

Preparation

Print out a copy of the worksheet for each student and have access to a flip chart/whiteboard/
A3 paper.

Instructions

- The group leader gives each group member their own mind map and asks them to write
  down as many jobs as they can.

- When they have finished this, the students provide their answers and the group leader
  writes these down on the flip chart. The group leader should place certain jobs in categories
  (e.g. doctors and nurses in medical, or carpenter or builder in construction). The group can
  then discuss why these are grouped similarly.

- After, students should choose three jobs which appeal and feel realistic to them, and write
  them down on their worksheet. They should then share these with the group and discuss
  why they think this would be a good job.

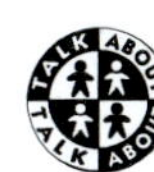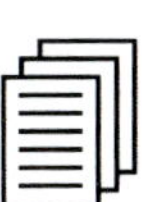

Activity 11 Jobs

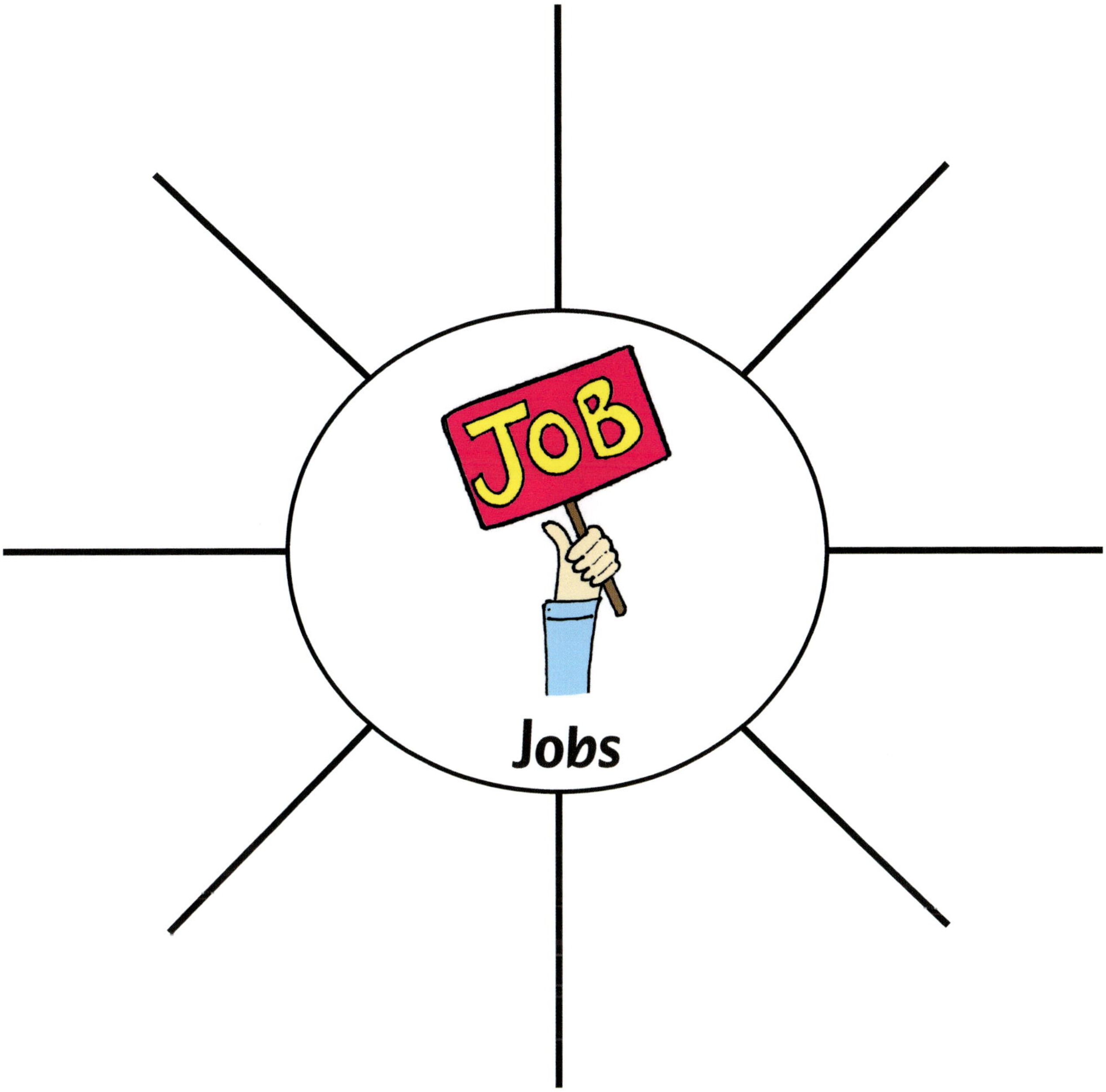

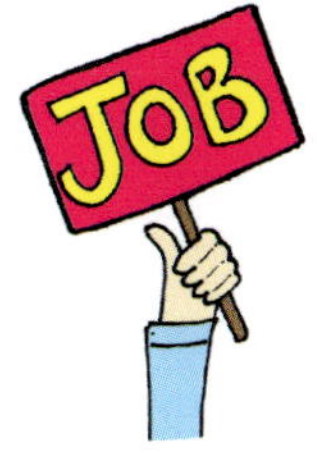

Three jobs that I think I can do and that sound good:

1. ....

2. ....

3. ....

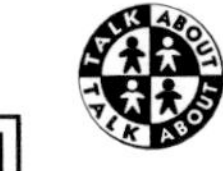
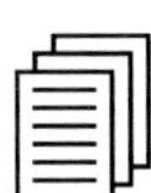

Activity 12 Choosing a job

Preparation

The group members will need their advert from Activity 7 and their jobs sheet from Activity 12. Print off a copy of the worksheet for each group member.

Instructions

- Encourage the group members to recap and share the information from their adverts.

- The group members go through the worksheet, identifying one interest, quality and skill that will help them carry out the first job on their list that they identified in the last session. They can also add new interests, qualities or skills if they would like to.

- After this, the group members can identify one skill that they could work on to support them to carry out the jobs they've identified.

- If they have enough time, they could do the same thing for the other jobs they identified with a new worksheet.

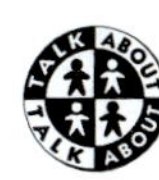

Activity 12 Choosing a job

One job I chose was:

....

....

One interest I have that will help me do this job is:

....

because this will help me ....

....

One skill I have that will help me do this job is:

....

because this will help me ....

....

One quality I have that will help do this job is:

....

because this will help me ....

....

One skill or quality I need to learn or develop is:

....

because this will help me ....

....

Activity 13 How do we get there?

Preparation

Group leaders can either reuse the occupation cards from Activity 10 and print out the large cards on the next page or print out the 'How do we get there?' worksheet for each group member. Group members will also need their worksheet from Activity 11.

Instructions

- First, the group leader introduces the words 'college', 'university', 'apprenticeship' and 'volunteering/work experience'. The group should then discuss what each of these means. Let the group know that each of these is a different route to getting a job.

- The first way to carry out this activity is to have the occupation cards in the middle of the group and each group member takes it in turns to take a card from the pile. The group member decides which route they need to go down to do this job and states their reason why. The group can discuss if there is any other way to do this. Some of the occupations will have more than one way of getting there.

- The second way to carry out this activity is to give each of the group members the worksheet and ask them to draw lines to match up the occupation to the route.

- Once they have completed this, provide them with their list of three jobs that they completed in Activity 4. Which routes do they need to choose to do the jobs they are interested in?

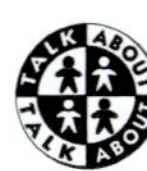
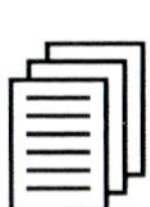

Activity 13 How do we get there?

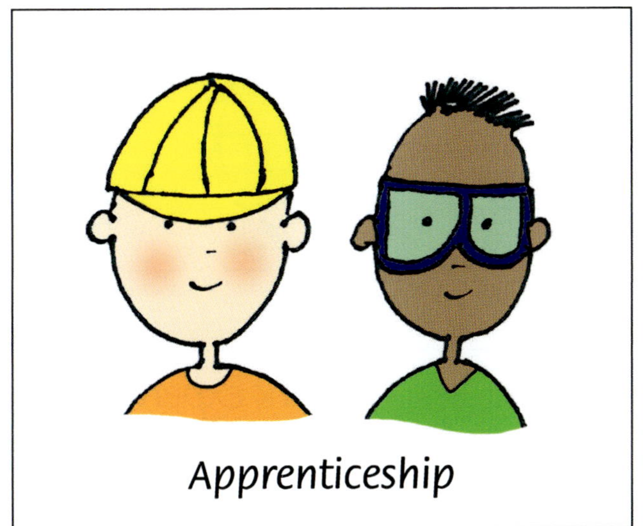

Apprenticeship

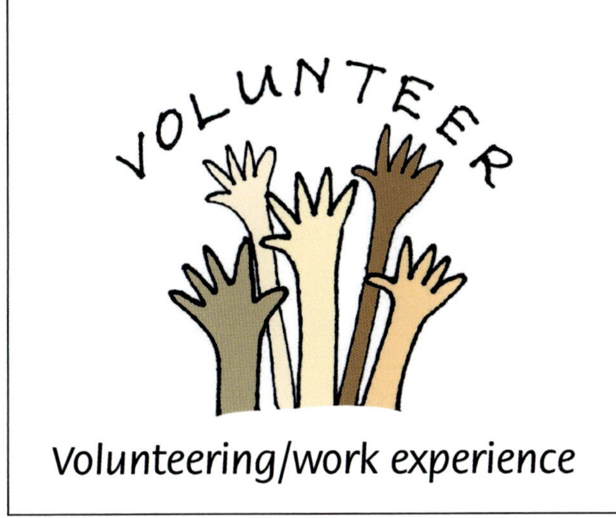

Volunteering/work experience

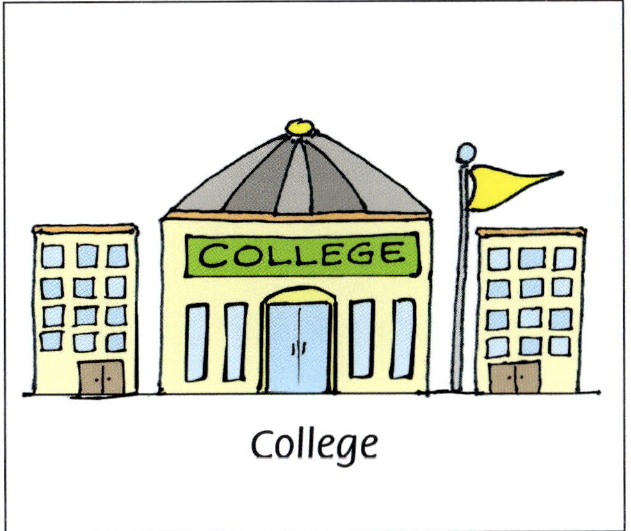

College

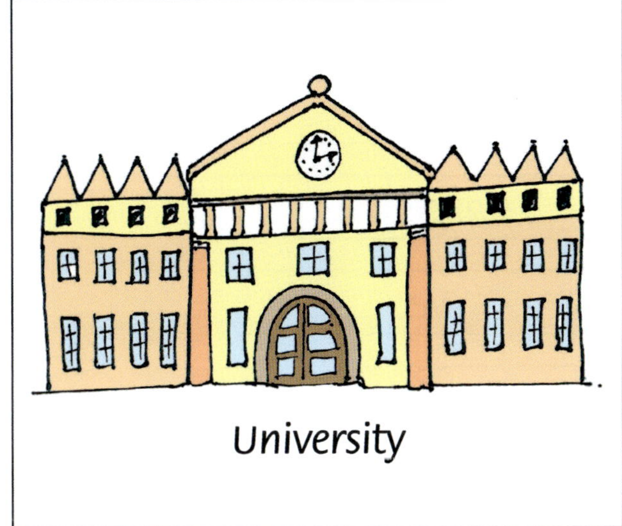

University

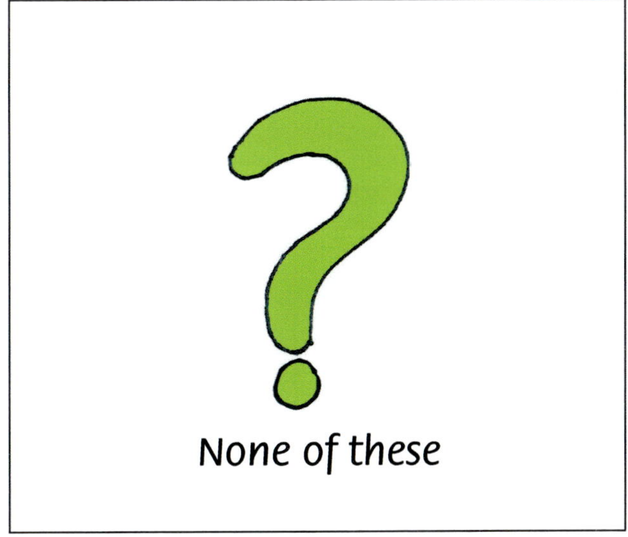

None of these

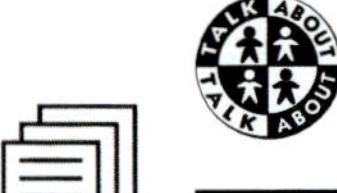

Activity 13 How do we get there?

| Teacher |
| Electrician |
| Builder |
| Chef |
| Dentist |
| Farmer |
| Nurse |
| Plumber |
| Carpenter |
| Vet |
| Gardener |
| Baker |
| Mechanic |
| Hairdresser |
| Police officer |
| Waiter/waitress |
| Taxi driver |
| Accountant |

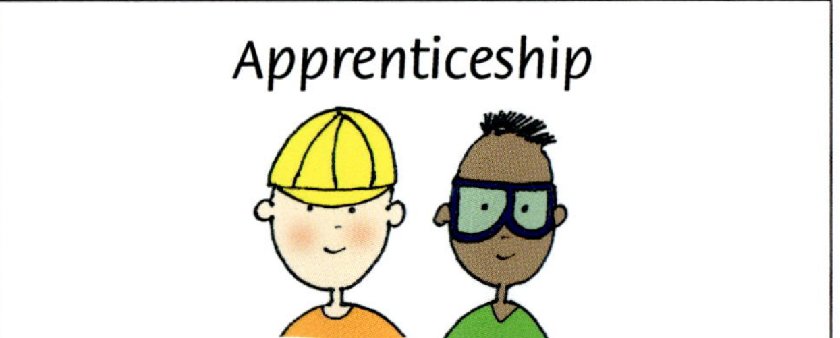
Apprenticeship

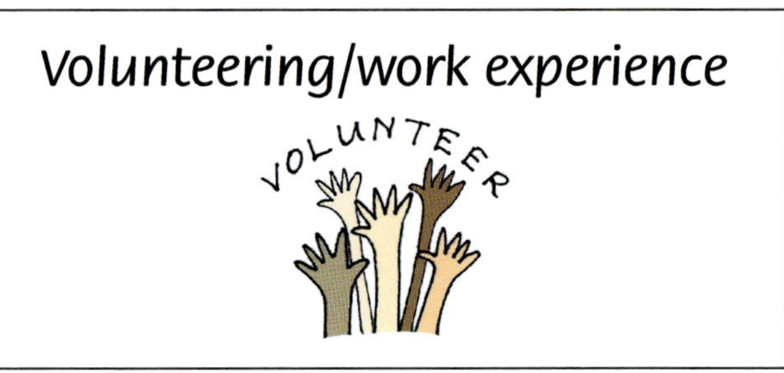
Volunteering/work experience

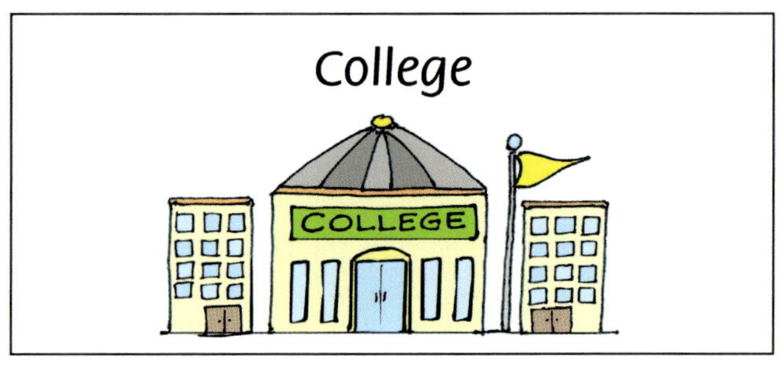
College

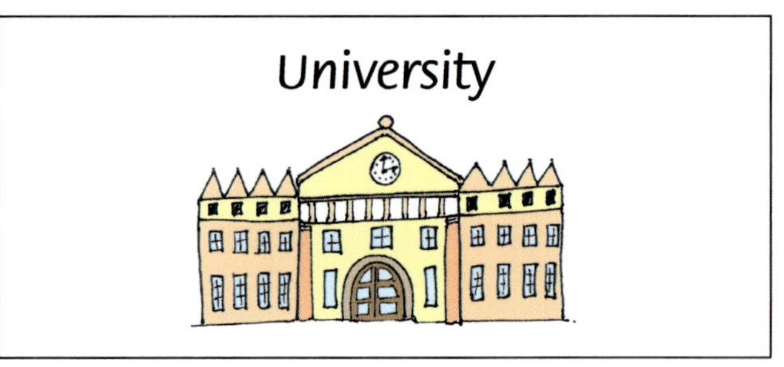
University

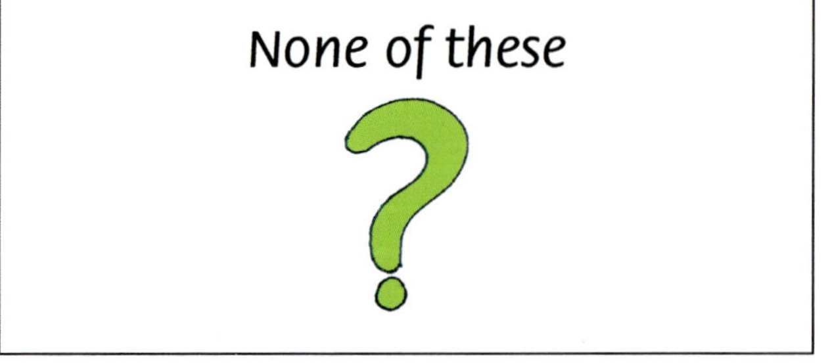
None of these

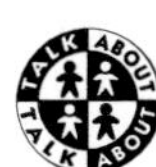
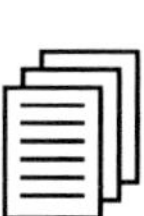

Activity 14 Which route do I take?

Preparation

Print out a copy of the worksheet for each route and provide all of these to each group member. It will be beneficial to have access to the internet for research purposes in this activity.

Instructions

- Group members are asked to read through the scenario for each route in pairs.

- After each scenario they should research the answers to the questions for each possible route and complete the worksheets. They can then complete a table indicating the positives and negatives of this route.

Activity 14 Which route do I take?

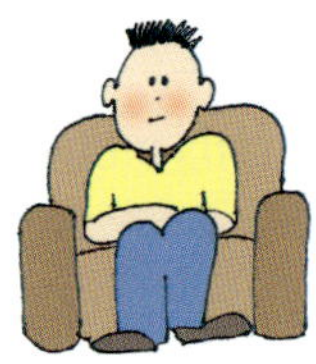

Mike left college three months ago and hasn't worked since. He wants to work in a school but can't seem to get an interview. Mike goes to the job centre every fortnight to claim unemployment benefit.

What does it mean to claim unemployment benefit?

....

How much will you be paid?

....

Where do you go to claim unemployment benefit?

....

Unemployment benefit	
Positives	**Difficulties**

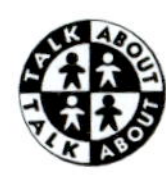
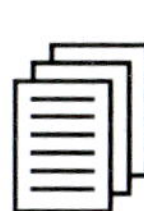

Activity 14 Which route do I take?

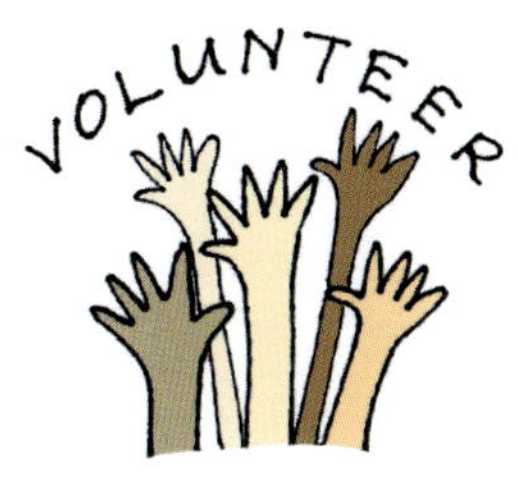

Trudie has not been able to get a job even though she's been to lots of interviews. All the people that have interviewed her have told her that she needs to get more experience in the field she's interested in.

What does volunteering mean?

....

What does work experience mean?

....

How much will you be paid?

....

Where can you go in your local area to find work experience or a place to volunteer?

....

Volunteering/work experience	
Positives	**Difficulties**

Activity 14 Which route do I take?

 After leaving school, Daniel didn't want to go to college or university and much preferred the practical subjects at his school like design technology and art. He applies for an apprenticeship.

What is an apprenticeship?

....

How much will you be paid?

....

Where can you be an apprentice?

....

Apprenticeships	
Positives	**Difficulties**

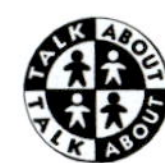

Activity 14 Which route do I take?

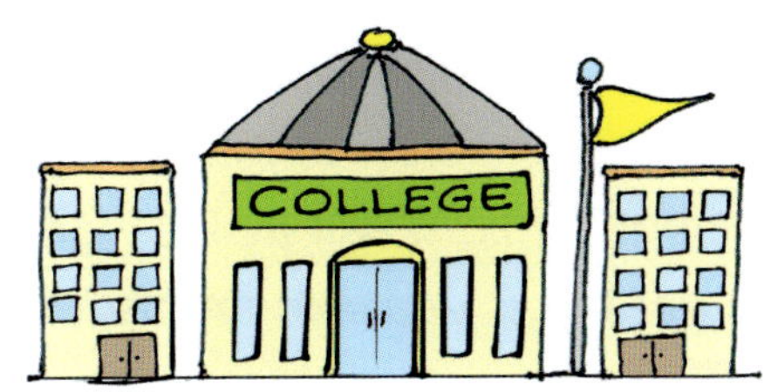

Ellie managed to get seven GCSE grades above a C and is thinking about going to college. She's been to look around her local college and her school sixth form and isn't sure which one to choose.

What is college?

....

What is sixth form?

....

How much will you be paid? How much do you have to pay?

....

What colleges or sixth forms are local to you?

....

College/sixth form	
Positives	**Difficulties**

Activity 14 Which route do I take?

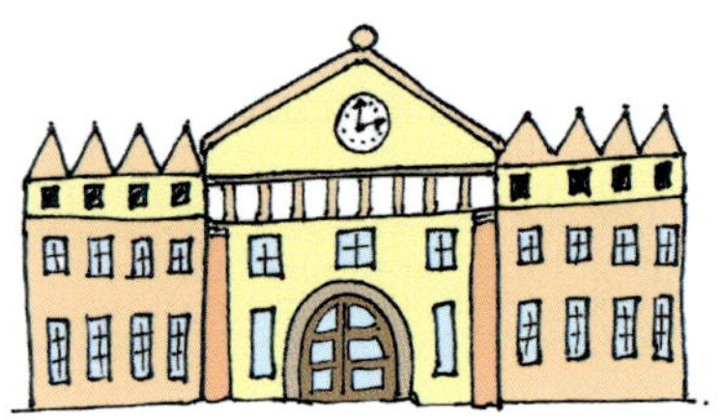

Nick has completed his A-levels and is waiting for his results over the summer. He has a place at a university quite far away from his home but thinks it will be best for his job prospects. He'd like to go, but it depends on his final grades.

What is university?

....

How much will you be paid? How much do you have to pay?

....

What universities are local to you?

....

University	
Positives	**Difficulties**

Activity 15 Next steps

Preparation

Print out a copy of the worksheet for each of the group members.

Instructions

- Let the group members know that they will be thinking about the jobs they identified in Activities 11 and 12 and how to get them.

- The group members should fill in each part of it, deciding what they need to do to be able to get to their job of choice.

- If the group members finish with enough time left, they can do another worksheet for another one of their selected jobs.

Activity 15 Next steps

| ✓ | **One of the jobs I chose was a** .... |

Do I need to do anything extra to do this job?

☐ Yes ← → No ☐

What do I have to do?

☐ College   ☐ Apprenticeship

☐ University   ☐ Work experience

☐ Volunteering   ☐ Other

Next steps

....

....

....

Topic 3 – Application process

Objectives   To understand what makes a good CV.

To create a CV using the provided template.

To become familiar with covering letters and application forms, and choose some references.

To know where to look for jobs.

Timing   This topic will take up to seven sessions to complete.

Activity	Description
Will I get an interview? (Activity 16)	Group members look at four CVs and decide what is good and what is bad about each one.
Help me out! (Activity 17)	Group members cut out and rearrange a jumbled up CV and discuss how to create a CV.
Writing a CV (Activity 18)	Group members use a template to create the answers for their own CV and then write these up into a digital CV.
Covering letters (Activity 19)	The group members fill in the blank words for a covering letter.
Application forms and references (Activity 20)	Each group member chooses a job to apply for and then fills in an application form for this job. They then discuss who would be appropriate to use as a reference in an application form.
Personal statement (Activity 21)	This exercise is optional depending on whether the group are thinking about university. The group members discuss the guidelines for personal statements and fill in a mind map with the relevant information.
Looking for a job (Activity 22)	The group members discuss and research where jobs can be found and then work through some short case studies.
Timeline (Activity 23)	The group members organise a timeline of steps from applying for a job to waiting to find out about a job.

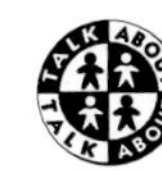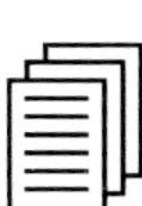

Activity 16 Will I get an interview?

Preparation

Photocopy the CVs for each group member. Photocopy the table or enlarge it to A3 (or use a flipchart/whiteboard).

Instructions

- Tell the group that in this session they will be in charge of deciding whether someone is going to get an interview. Explain that they will be looking at four different people's CV and deciding what is good and what is bad about them. Hand out the four CVs to each group member.

- Explain what a CV is – an advert of someone's skills and readiness to carry out a job, including their qualifications, education, work experience and personality. Some studies say that employers will look at a CV for up to about 20 seconds, but on average it will be six seconds!

- Look through one CV at a time and read out the information to the group. Encourage the group members to make notes on parts of it that they think are good or bad, including what the person is saying in their CV and how it is laid out.

- Once they have finished one CV, encourage group discussion around what makes a good CV and what makes a bad CV. Use the table in this activity (or write a table on the board or flipchart) to create a list for each side. Who are they going to give an interview to?

Activity 16 Will I get an interview?

CV – Jennifer Woods

Address: 78 Shepton Drive, GIVESWORTH, SHOMPSHIRE, YS7 6AB
Tel: 07888 889546   Email: coolcargirl@yahoo.co.uk
DoB: 18th October 1993   Nationality: British
Gender: Female   Marital status: Single (and ready to mingle!)

Personal profile

I have worked in lots of different businesses over the last few years. I work hard at work and like people on my team. I would like to contribute my skills to a business as I feel I am qualified for anything.

Education

1990–1996: Vale of Hadrian Primary School
1996–2001: Sherpington Manor Secondary School – 6 GCSEs
2001–2003: A-levels at Givesworth College
- English B
- Theatre Studies C
- Psychology D
2003–2006: University College Birmingham – BSc Psychology

Work

2011–Present	Computer support	Jade Computer Solutions
2008–2011	Administration	Wright & Gray Legal Firm
2006–2008	Sales assistant	KBP Auto Vehicle Sales Group

Hobbies and interests

I really love going on holiday, playing football, eating meals and going for cycle rides.

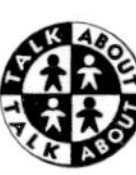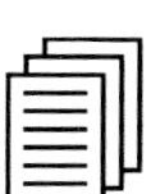

Activity 16 Will I get an interview?

Curriculum Vitae – Ava Chowdhury

18 Trutton Drive, Meedon, ME66 8RB
Mob: 07954 214589   Email: ava.chowdhury@gmail.com

Personal profile

I am a flexible, enthusiastic and hard-working graduate student. I am seeking a position in the translation department of a business where I can use the problem-solving and language skills I have developed through university and employment.

Education

2006–2010 – French and German (BA Hons)
• Solus Town University, with year abroad in Bern, Switzerland

2004–2006 – A-levels   St John's Secondary School
• English – B
• French – B
• German – C

1999–2004 – 8 GCSEs A*–C   St John's Secondary School
• English – B   • German – B
• Maths – C   • Science – C
• French – C   • ICT – C

Work

2013–Present   Translator for German language at GR Sports

I worked with various suppliers, distributors and retail outlets to ensure trusted relationships were built and orders delivered efficiently. This involved communicating both by phone and email, as well as organising and managing time and travel effectively for individual clients. I regularly earned positive feedback as a team member for being proactive and knowledgeable.

2010–2013   Translator for French language version of MGW magazine

I was entrusted with the translation of various articles centred around sport, fashion and business and developed various presentations to market the magazine to potential new customers in France. I worked with authors closely to ensure the translation was accurate and used Microsoft Word, Publisher and PowerPoint on a daily basis.

Hobbies and interests

I enjoy socialising, travelling and swimming and I volunteer at a local charity shop every Saturday morning.

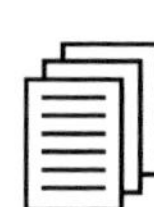
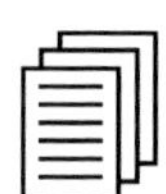

Activity 16 Will I get an interview?

ANDY

18 GRABBAN ROAD, RHY-ON-WEAR, RO4 1EF
MOB: 07895 545978   EMAIL: BADBOY43@GMAIL.COM

PERSONAL STUFF

READY TO GO OUT TO WORK AND EARN SOME MONEY FOR A NEW TV. I SOMETIMES ARGUE WITH PEOPLE BUT IT'S ONLY BECAUSE I'M RIGHT ABOUT EVERYTHING. I'M INTERESTED IN DOING A JOB THAT I GET TO CHOOSE MY HOURS AND GO IN LATE BECAUSE I LOVE SLEEPING IN.

EDUCATION

BTEC COLLEGE LEVEL 2 CONSTRUCTION
FUNCTIONAL SKILLS LEVEL 3
SOME GCSES

WORK

HAVEN'T WORKED BEFORE BUT I DID DO SOME WORK EXPERIENCE AT MY DAD'S CAR WAREHOUSE. I DID A LOT OF LIFTING AND MOVING STUFF AND LOVED GETTING ON THE FORKLIFT TRUCK TO DRIVE AROUND THE WAREHOUSE.

HOBBIES AND INTERESTS

I LOVE GOING OUT AT THE WEEKEND WITH MY MATES.

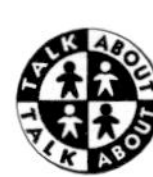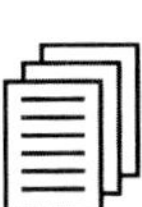

Activity 16 Will I get an interview?

Sam Shao – Curriculum Vitae

84 Lockington Crescent, Southampton, SO58 7DU

samshao10@businessmail.com   – 01564 965 841 – 07764 184 930

Personal statement

I am a responsible and hard-working employee looking for a job where I will be able to use skills that I have learnt in college and on work experience. I am able to be flexible and work in a team.

Education and qualifications

Moor Dock College

BTEC Level 2 Diploma in Construction – modules covered included:

- Construction and contracting operations
- Surveying and property maintenance
- Building environment design
- Health, safety and welfare in the built environment

Sherpington High School – GCSEs

- English – C
- Maths – C
- Science – D
- ICT – D
- PE – D
- Citizenship – E

Employment history and work experience

Griffin's Painting and Decorating – January 2015–July 2016

- Every Saturday I worked with a partner on using different painting techniques and wallpapering skills in houses, flats and office buildings. I understand the different health and safety standards that are required.
- I am able to measure accurately and prepare surfaces.
- I have used a variety of materials, including plaster, metal and wood to improve many building types, including offices.
- I am aware of various ways to use technology in the design of a room and paint mixing.
- I am familiar with specialist approaches, like rag rolling and marbling.

Pizza House – Back of house staff – December 2013–January 2015

- I worked in a team to provide a quality food service in the kitchen of a restaurant.

Hobbies and interests

I enjoy extreme sports and take part in skateboarding competitions regularly.

Activity 16 Will I get an interview?

Describe the good and bad things that you see in the CVs.

✔ Good	✘ Bad

Activity 17 Help me out!

Preparation

Photocopy the worksheets and the guidelines for each group member. They will also need a pair of scissors and a blank piece of A4 paper. Alternatively, if you'd like to carry this out as a group, print out the worksheet in A3 and place a blank sheet of A3 paper in the middle of the group (or on a flipchart).

Instructions

- Explain to the group that today they will be making sure they are able to organise a CV in the right order by helping someone put their CV together. Ask the group members to cut out the different parts of the CV and encourage them to place them in the order that they believe is correct, based on what they can remember from the last activity. After this, they can glue them onto the blank sheet of A4.

- The headings should follow this structure:
  - Curriculum vitae – name
  - Personal information
  - Personal profile
  - Education
  - Work
  - Hobbies

- After they have completed this, look through the worksheet that includes the guidelines for a CV and encourage discussion around these points.

Activity 17 Help me out!

Sales Assistant, ShopTop – June 2012–October 2014
I worked within a team to ensure that we regularly achieved a profit in the shop over every monthly period that I worked there. I am aware of how to operate a standard checkout till, carry out a stock check and organise a delivery.

2008–2010 – GCSE – Brockstable Secondary School

- English – C
- Maths – C
- Media – C

- Art – B
- Spanish – C
- Double Science – DD

Hobbies

Digital Camera Specialist, Costins – October 2014–Present
In this role, I employ knowledge of the specialist product which is on offer and provide advice and guidance to customers depending on their needs. I have reached my sales targets in each of my last 12 months and have worked with the management team to carry out leadership training.

Personal profile

Mateo Woźniak — Curriculum Vitae

I regularly go to the gym and enjoy keeping fit and healthy. I am a keen photographer and attend photography events at local galleries.

Education and qualifications

19 Private Drive, Shalder, Kent, CT39 1KK
Home phone: 04958 104954 Mobile: 07439 392194 Email: mateo.wozniak@email.com

Work

I am a responsible, focused and eager individual with experience in sales at a variety of companies. I work well in a team and have good interpersonal skills with customers. I regularly reach and exceed targets in my sales roles.

2010–2012 – A levels – Brockstable Sixth Form College
French – C   Media Studies – C   Chemistry – D

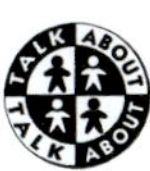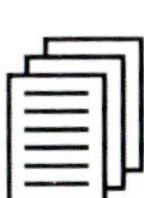

Activity 17 Help me out!

Guidelines for writing a CV

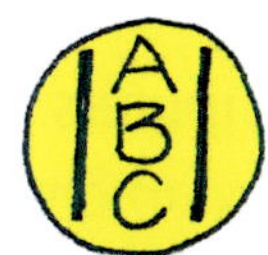

Keep to a structure

This will make it easy to read! Use the following headings:

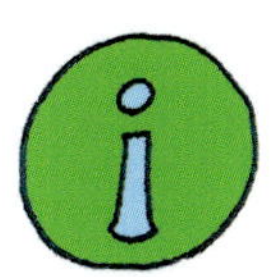

Personal information

Be sure to include your contact details (and make sure your email address is professional!). There's no need to include your date of birth, gender or nationality.

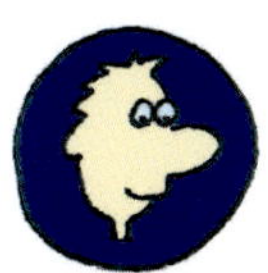

Personal profile

Explain your current situation (e.g. you're doing GCSEs/work part-time), use your qualities to advertise yourself and explain what opportunity you're looking for.

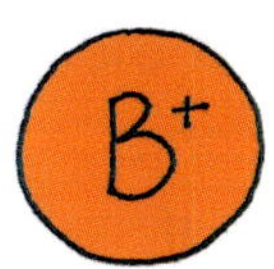

Education and qualifications

Start with your most recent first. Include where you studied and what you studied. Don't list all your GCSEs, but select a sample. (If you haven't done any GCSEs yet, list the subjects you're taking and when you're taking them.) Don't lie about these!

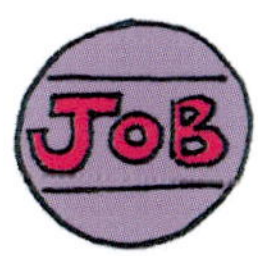

Employment

Again, start with your most recent job first, explaining where you worked and what you did – include three key skills that you used at this job. You can also include work experience and voluntary work in this part.

Hobbies/interests

Keep this section brief. Include a few relevant hobbies.

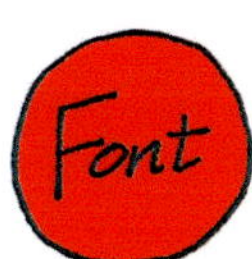

Format

- Make sure the font is clear and easy to read.
- Keep it brief and to the point – no longer than two pages.
- Before you send it out, make sure to check the spelling and grammar. Ask someone to check it for you before you send it off.

Activity 18 Writing a CV

Preparation

Provide the group with the CV template from the following worksheet. The group will be required to have digital copies of this, so alternatively, if the group is able to access computers or laptops for the following session, the group leaders could create the template in a document using the headings on the next page that everyone can access. The group can then type their ideas directly into this. If not, it is recommended that the group leaders type up their answers from the written documents so that the group members have their own individual CVs to take away after this programme.

Instructions

- Explain to the group that, after looking at other people's CVs and the guidelines for creating a CV, they will be creating their own CVs today.

- Provide them with the template on the following worksheet (or on a document on the computer) and ask them to fill as many parts as they can with support from you and the guidelines discussed last week. Encourage them to think back to previous topics to come up with answers, for example they have already listed their qualities back in Topic 1. If appropriate, use the examples of good CVs from Activity 1 in this topic to show what kind of language is expected in a CV.

- Once they have completed their CVs, print the individual CVs out for the group members and keep them in a safe place that they can access when needed.

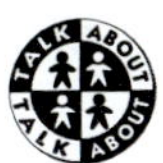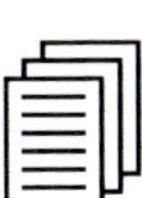

Activity 18 Writing a CV

Personal information

Name:
Address:
Phone number:
Email address:

Personal profile

What are you doing at the moment? (e.g. GCSEs, A-levels, college course)

....

What three important qualities do you have? (e.g. hard-working, reliable)

....

What kind of work are you looking for?

....

Education and qualifications

Where do you go to school/college?

....

What qualifications do you have? Or are you completing them now? (Put the most recent first.)

....

Employment

Have you worked anywhere? Have you volunteered/had any work experience? (Put the most recent first.)

....

....

....

Hobbies/interests

List three hobbies or interests that you have.

....

....

Activity 19 Covering letters

Preparation

Photocopy the worksheet.

Instructions

- Discuss the importance of a covering letter. It introduces who you are and provides group members with an opportunity to show how enthusiastic they are for a job.

- Group members can complete the worksheet by filling in the gaps with the correct words or use their own words to fill in the gaps.

- Once they have completed this, ensure that group members are aware that this example is very generic – if they are to use this as a covering letter, they may need to add more specific items related to the company they are looking at working for.

- To extend this activity, the group members can write out a covering letter for themselves for a specific job.

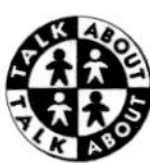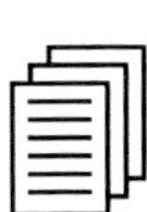

Activity 19 Covering letters

Jake Musing
60 Lockington Crescent
Southampton
SO58 7DU

Mr Griffin
Griffin's Painting and Decorating
18 Nursford Road
Southampton
SO23 4OT

Dear_____________,

I am writing to enquire about any job _____________ or opportunities within your _____________, Griffin's Painting and Decorating.

Please find attached a copy of my CV. I am currently completing a BTEC level 2 Diploma in _____________ and am _____________ about using my current learning practically. I am _____________, reliable and determined in my work and I feel that this would make me the _____________ candidate for a role with your company.

I am committed to providing a _____________ service in whatever environment I work in and would enjoy _____________ more from people who are extremely _____________ in this field.

Thank you for taking the _____________ to read this email.

Yours _____________,

Jake Musing

Use the following words to complete the letter:

hard-working	perfect	enthusiastic	vacancies
time	experienced	Mr Griffin	Construction
high quality	company	sincerely	learning

Activity 20 Application forms and references

Preparation

Photocopy the job descriptions list and the application form. Alternatively, if computer or laptop access is available, find digital application forms for real jobs and see if the group members can fill these in instead.

Instructions

- Tell the group members that over one third of all jobs require them to fill in a job application instead of writing out a CV. They can use their CVs and previous qualities work to complete the application form. They should try to make it relevant to the job description as well.

- Once they get to the second page, they will be required to write down references. Before they do this, provide them with the references worksheet. Discuss what a reference is – someone that employers refer to so that they can find out if the person that applied for a job will be someone they want to work with. Employers will talk to referees once they have interviewed someone.

- Once they have completed the worksheet, discuss why the people they have ticked make good references and who they could include as their own reference. They could then include these on their application form.

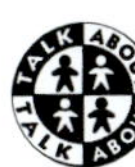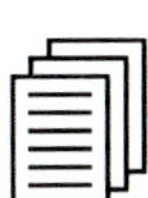

Activity 20 Application forms

Choose your job and companies for the application forms. The following are the job responsibilities of...

A receptionist at Jersey Office Towers

Greet visitors in person or by phone. Answer questions or connect to other people in the company who can help. Show visitors where to go in the building. Keep employee and department records up to date on the computer system.

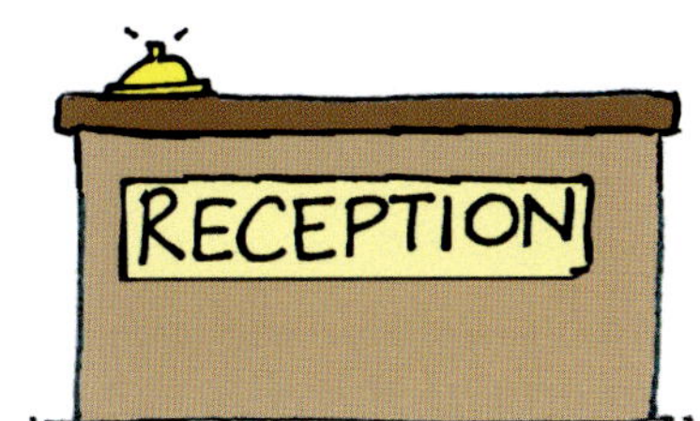

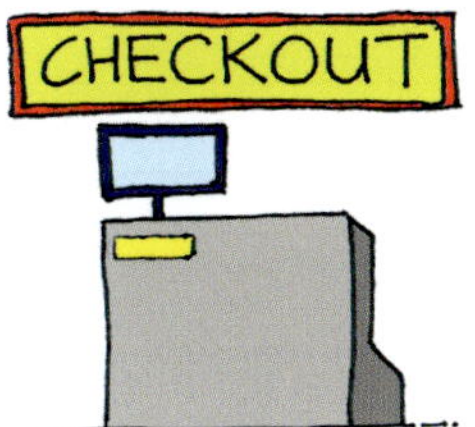

A retail store salesperson at Mixpo Electronics

Help customers select products and use a checkout till. Interact well with customers and learn about the relevant electronic products. Work in a team.

A food server at Roasties Dining

Take orders and serve food and drink to customers at tables in a restaurant. Make sure customers are enjoying their meals and help them if they need anything else.

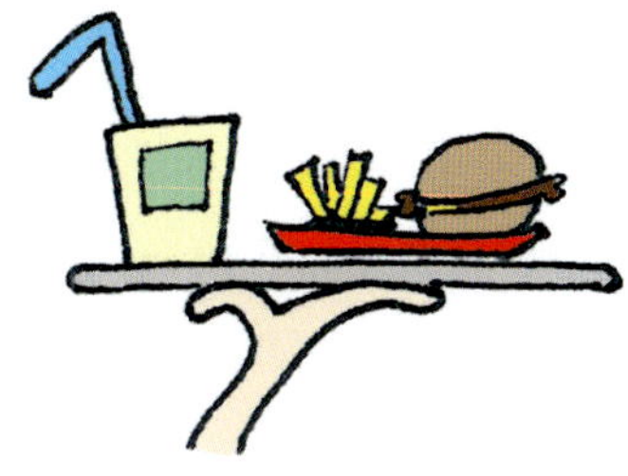

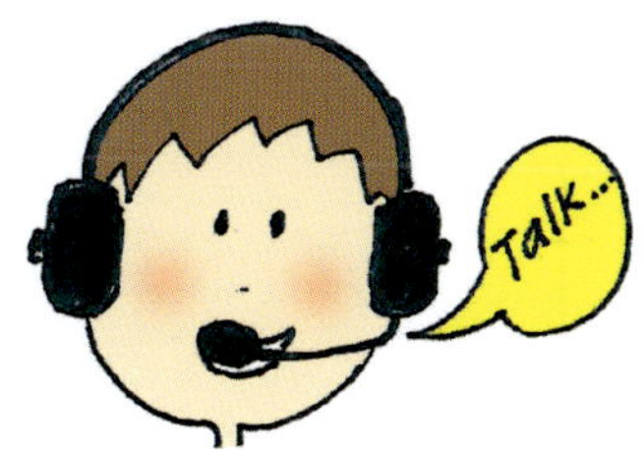

A call centre worker at GG Phones

Figure out what is wrong with customers' phones or the network. Answer questions about the service and solve problems. Use a computer to fill in a database.

A mechanic at SuperWheels

Inspect, fix and maintain vehicles. Problem-solve by looking at vehicles and answer questions about the work. Follow instructions and health and safety procedures.

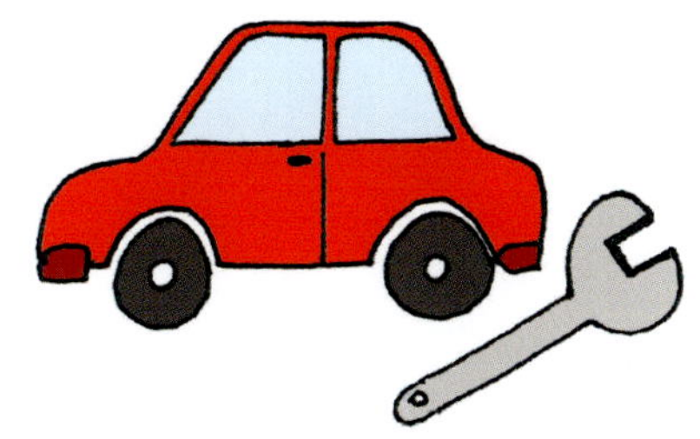

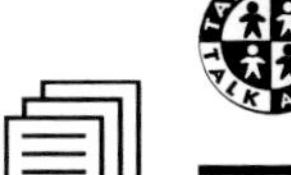
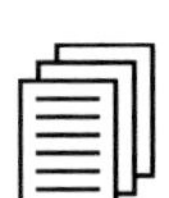

Activity 20 Application forms

Job application form

About the vacancy
Vacancy applied for: ____
Employer's name: ____
Closing date: _______ /_______ /_______

Personal details
Title: Mr   Mrs   Miss   Ms   Other
Surname: ____
Other names: ____
Address: ____

____

____

Daytime phone number: ____
Mobile phone number: ____
Email address: ____
Driving licence held?   Yes   No

Work history
Start with your most recent job and work back. Continue on a separate sheet if necessary.

Employer	Position held and description of duties	Reason for leaving

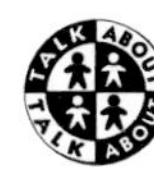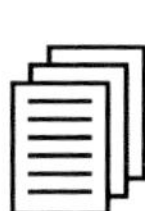

Activity 20 Application forms

Education and training

Start with your most recent education and work back. Continue on a separate sheet if necessary.

University, college, school or other place	Course studied and qualifications achieved

Any other evidence

In this section, include any experience that is relevant to the job you are applying for.

References

1. Name:	2. Name:
_____________________________	_____________________________
Relationship:	Relationship:
_____________________________	_____________________________
Phone number:	Phone number:
_____________________________	_____________________________
Occupation:	Occupation:

I confirm that, to the best of my knowledge, the information I have given on this form is correct.

Signature: _____________________________ Date: _______ / _______ / _______

Activity 20 References

Who makes a good reference?

Put a tick next to the people you think would make good references. ☑

Grandma: 'Oh, he's such a good boy, stays out of trouble and makes a lovely cup of tea.' ☐

Teacher: 'She worked hard in all her classes, independently and in groups, and no other teacher had a bad word to say about her.' ☐

Dad: 'He's a great lad, doesn't complain when things go wrong and is really level-headed.' ☐

Boss: 'He's been dedicated to providing a really high level of work since he started and is always really keen to learn new things.' ☐

Friend: 'She's always up for a laugh and is really determined – never wants to give up an argument.' ☐

Neighbour: 'She was always very helpful during the summer, working in our garden to keep it tidy every Saturday.' ☐

Work experience supervisor: 'He was really enthusiastic and was a positive influence on the team, really pushed them forward in difficult moments.' ☐

A famous person you have a signed photo of: 'Eh? Who am I giving a reference for? I don't even know him!' ☐

Who could your references be? Pick up to two people from your life:

Reference 1:

....

Reference 2:

....

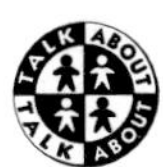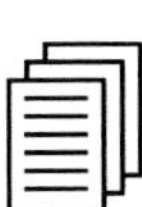

Activity 21 Personal statement

Preparation

This activity is optional depending on whether the group members are or will be in the process of applying for university. For this activity, photocopy the general guidelines for writing a personal statement and the mind map for each group member.

Instructions

- Go through the guidelines with the group members. Encourage discussion around what could go into each area.

- Provide each group member with a copy of the mind map. They can fill this in with notes that they feel are relevant to their application to university.

Activity 21 Personal statement

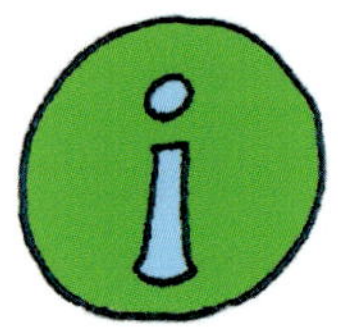

General guidelines for writing a personal statement

- It can be up to 4,000 characters or 47 lines long.

- Make it original – it's **your** personal statement, not anyone else's!

- You can only write one statement, so don't write to one university specifically.

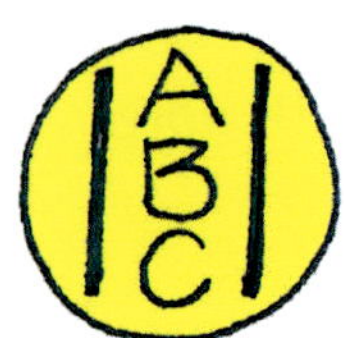

- Use a **structure**, like the following:

  o **Introduction** – Begin with a paragraph that shows your enthusiasm and makes the person reading want to continue.

  o **Main body** – This is where you put in what is relevant for the universities you're applying for.

  o **Conclusion** – Restate the main skills or qualities that would be useful for the course you're applying for. Emphasise your enthusiasm for it.

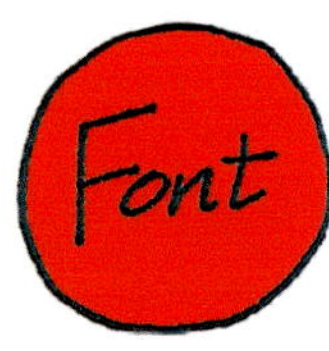

- Before you send it out, make sure to check the **spelling and grammar**. Get someone to check it for you and if necessary, rewrite it.

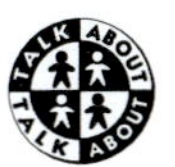
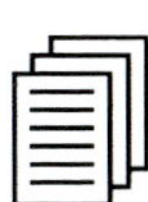

Activity 21 Personal statement

The course I am applying for is ....

What activities or hobbies do you do that are relevant to this course?

What skills or qualities do you have that are relevant to this course?

Why are you interested in this subject?

What is relevant about your previous jobs, placement or work experiences to the course?

Activity 22 Looking for a job

Preparation

Enlarge the mind map to A3 or draw it out on a flipchart. Photocopy the worksheet.

Instructions

- Before handing out the worksheets, encourage discussion between pairs around where we find jobs. Where do the group members think that they can look for jobs? These will include newspapers, the internet (specific websites if appropriate), job centre, friends and family contacts, and going to places to drop off CVs. Ask them to give feedback and write these up on the mind map. The group leaders may have to provide prompts or supplement the group members' knowledge if they're not sure.

- Once there is a variety of places to look for jobs on the mind map, provide each pair with one of the scenarios. Ask them to go through the questions and answer them. If possible, provide the group members with research time on the internet or real life examples of job sections in newspapers, specific websites, etc.

- Once every pair is finished, ask each group to give feedback about their scenario and what their plan for the person would be. Encourage discussion amongst the other group members – do they think this is the right career to do, or the right place to be looking?

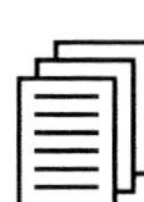

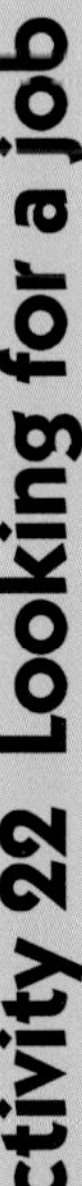

Activity 22 Looking for a job

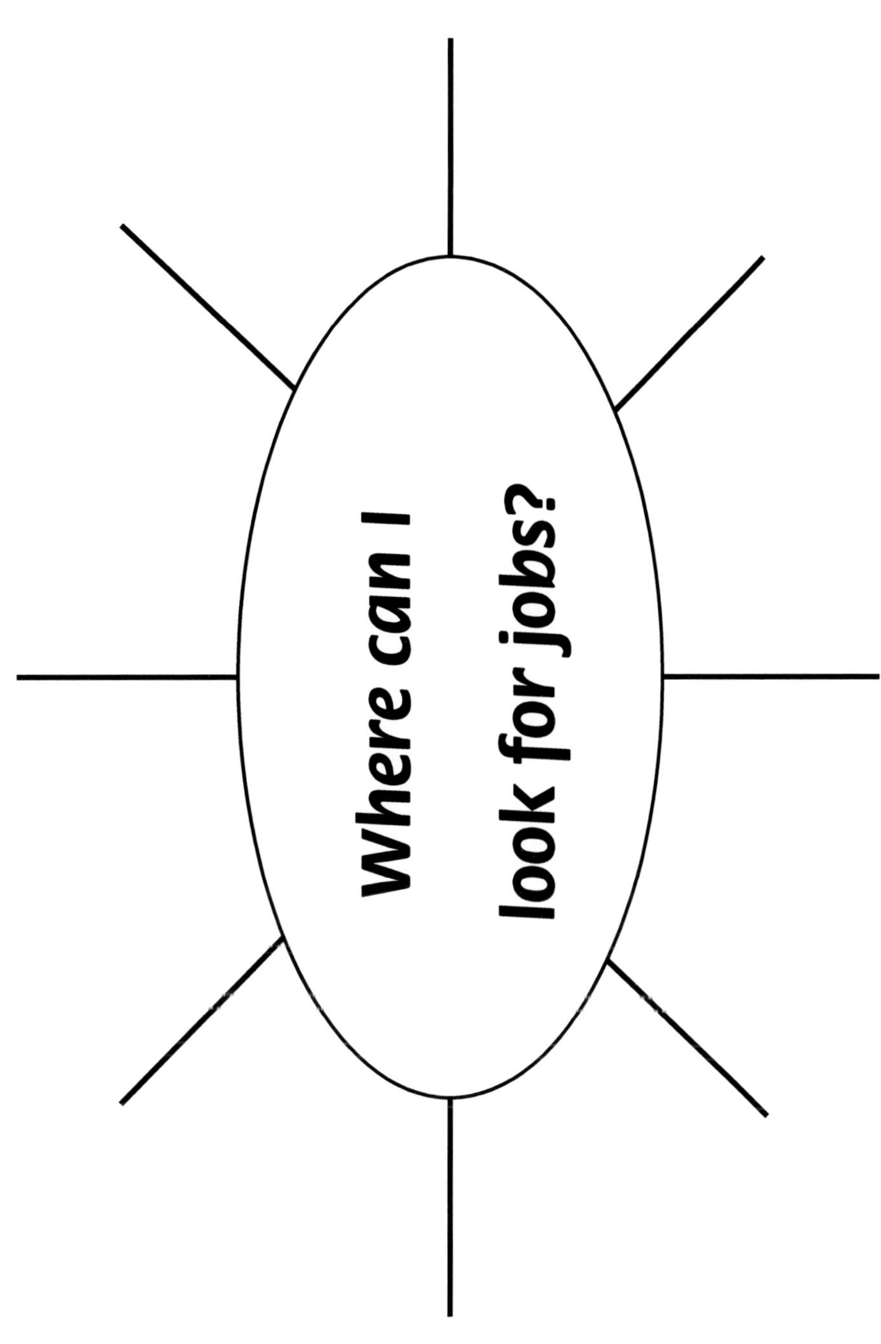

Where can I look for jobs?

Activity 22 Looking for a job

Adam has just finished a qualification in catering. He enjoys working in restaurant kitchens but would also like to try being part of the waiting staff. He has a Saturday job in his uncle's restaurant.

Where do you think Adam could work?

....

What else could Adam do to help him with working there?

....

Where should Adam go to find jobs?

....

Amar hates working in her current job because there isn't any chance of a promotion. Amar has a degree in Computing and would like to put this to use.

Where do you think Amar could work?

....

What else could Amar do to help her with working there?

....

Where should Amar go to find jobs?

....

Hope works in a supermarket but wants to be able to earn more money. She is very chatty and friendly and feels like she would be good in a sales role.

Where do you think Hope could work?

....

What else could Hope do to help her with working there?

....

Where should Hope go to find jobs?

....

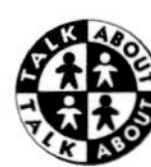
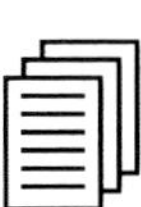

Activity 23 Timeline

Preparation

Enlarge the timeline sheet to A3 or draw the timeline on a flipchart or whiteboard. Photocopy, cut out and laminate the timeline cards.

Instructions

- If working in pairs or groups, ask the group members to take it in turns to pick a card and place it on the timeline where they think it should go. Encourage them to move other cards around if they think that they're in the wrong place.

- Make sure to discuss the time between everything – even though all the cards will be close together, there might be a lot of time between 'Send off my CV and covering letter/ application form' and 'Receive a reply inviting me to interview' but not a lot between 'Leave for interview with plenty of time to arrive at least ten minutes early' and 'Have the interview'.

Activity 23 Timeline

Place the cards where you think they go on the timeline.

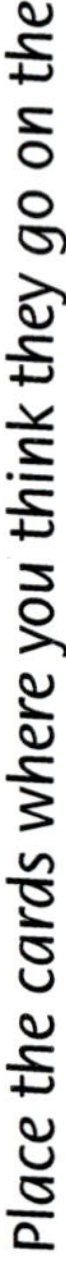

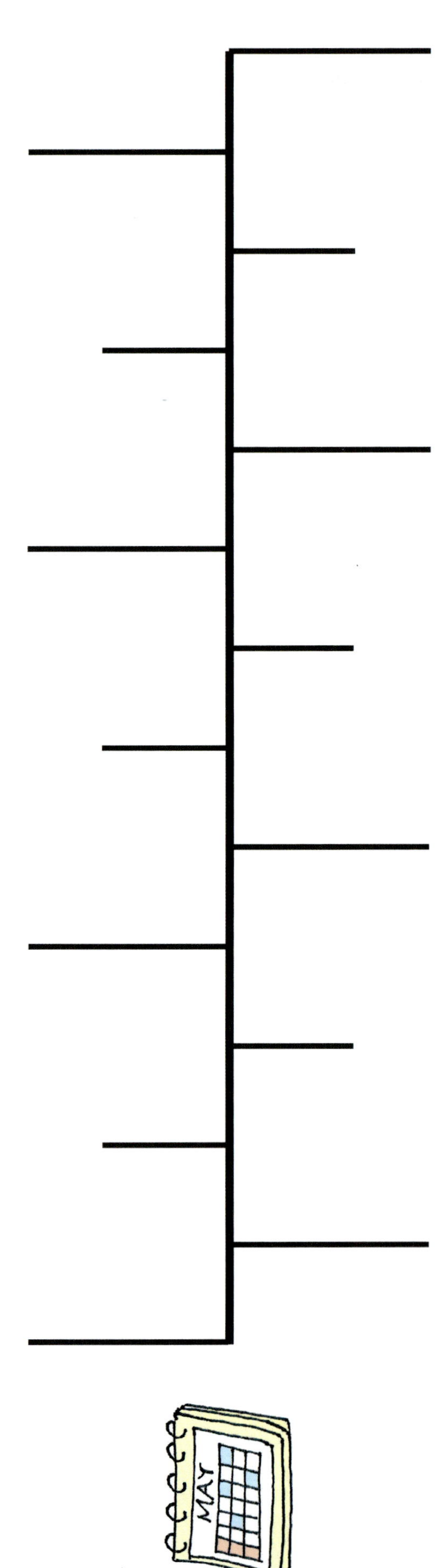

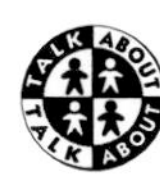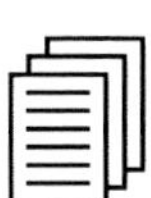

Activity 23 Timeline

Find a job that I think I might like	Receive a reply inviting me to interview
Decide what I'd like to do as a job	Wait to find out if I got the job
Wash and iron clothes suitable for interview	Send off my CV and covering letter/application form
Let the employers know that I'll be attending the interview	Write a CV
Remember to bring paperwork that employers might need to see	Write a covering letter or application form
Leave for interview with plenty of time to arrive early	Have the interview
Prepare for interview questions	Look for a job in newspapers, on the internet, etc.

Topic 4 – Interviews

Objectives

To prepare for and practise an interview for a job.

To understand the aspects of body language and the way we talk that are important during an interview.

To prepare answers to common interview questions.

To reflect on the performance during two interviews – one at the beginning of the topic and one at the end.

Timing

This topic will take up to ten sessions to complete.

TALKABOUT TRANSITIONS Interviews

Activity	Description
Interview (Activity 24)	The group members choose a job to interview for. They prepare answers to common questions and then reflect on their performance using an evaluation form. This may take up to two sessions to complete.
How do I look? (Activity 25)	The group members discuss what is appropriate and not appropriate to wear to an interview and discuss the rules around the relevant aspects of body language. This may take up to two sessions to complete.
How do I sound? (Activity 26)	The group leaders provide good and bad models of certain aspects of the way we talk and conversational skills and reflect on the rules to each one. This may take up to two sessions to complete.
Good and bad answers (Activity 27)	The group leaders model good and bad answers to common interview questions. The group reflect on the rules for each one.
Interview questions (Activity 28)	The group members create more detailed answers to the common interview questions.
Second interview (Activity 29)	The group members carry out another job interview using the skills they have learnt over the topic. They then reflect on their performance using the same evaluation form.
Comparing interviews (Activity 30)	The group compare their two evaluation forms from the beginning and the end of the topic. Have they improved? What could they still improve on?

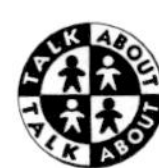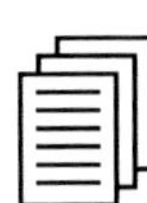

Activity 24 Interview

Preparation

Depending on how supportive you feel the other members of the group will be, this session may require one group leader to set up in a separate room to conduct interviews with each group member. In this room, you should use a video camera or mobile phone to record the group members' interviews for later comparison. Alternatively, if you feel that the group members can work together, they can work in pairs to interview each other. Ideally, the group members would be recorded still.

Photocopy either the group or individual evaluation forms. This activity may take up to two sessions.

Instructions

- Explain to the group that the following topic is going to look at the next stage of the process of getting a job or a college place, the interview. Let them know that they will take part in an interview and that all the activities in the next topic will look at how they can improve at their interviews.

- Once the group leaders have decided on the above process, provide each of the group members with the job descriptions sheet and ask them to choose a job to interview for.

- As soon as they know what job they would like to be interviewed for, the group members take it in turns to be interviewed and recorded. The group leader interviewing can use the script provided with the six questions.

- Whilst this is happening, it will be beneficial for the other group leader to run a different and fun activity to ensure the other group members do not experience anxiety and to enable the rest of the group to be engaged.

- When all the group members have had an interview, watch these together (if each group member is comfortable with this). The others should rate their performance and provide constructive criticism and possible improvements. Remind the group members that it's okay that their scores aren't perfect as they will be practising all these skills over the next sessions. If they would prefer to look at their own interview by themselves, use the individual rating scale provided.

- Keep these rating sheets until the last activity in this topic, a second interview for comparison.

Activity 24 Interview

Choose your job before the interview. The following are the job responsibilities of. . .

Receptionist: Greet visitors in person or by phone. Answer questions or connect to other people in the company who can help. Show visitors where to go. Keep employee and department records up to date.

Food server: Take orders and serve food and drink to customers at tables in a restaurant. Make sure customers are enjoying their meals and help them if they need anything else.

Call centre worker: Figure out what is wrong with customers' phones or the network. Answer questions about the service and solve problems. Use a computer to fill in a database.

Retail store salesperson: Help customers select products and use a checkout till. Interact well with customers and learn about the relevant electronic products. Work in a team.

Mechanic: Inspect, fix and maintain vehicles. Problem-solve by looking at vehicles and answer questions about the work. Follow instructions and health and safety procedures.

Teacher: Plan and deliver lessons. Work with other teachers in a department. Mark students' work. Go to parents' evenings. Run after school groups.

Office worker: Use a computer to maintain files and records. Answer the phone. Do basic finance tasks, like issue invoices. Sort incoming and outgoing mail. Make sure there's enough stationery in the office.

Activity 24 Interview

1. What can you tell me about yourself or your personality?

....

....

....

2. Can you tell me your three biggest strengths?

....

....

....

3. Can you tell me one weakness about yourself?

....

....

....

4. Why do you want to work here?

....

....

....

5. What experience or skills do you have that might help you do this job?

....

....

....

6. What do you enjoy doing in your spare time?

....

....

....

Activity 24 Interview – group rating scale

	Name:	Name:	Name:	Name:	Name: ....
Did the candidate greet the interviewer appropriately?	Yes No	Yes No	Yes No	Yes No	Yes No
How good is the candidate's eye contact?	1 2 3 4 5	1 2 3 4 5	1 2 3 4 5	1 2 3 4 5	1 2 3 4 5
How good is the candidate's posture?	1 2 3 4 5	1 2 3 4 5	1 2 3 4 5	1 2 3 4 5	1 2 3 4 5
How good is the candidate's ability to sit still?	1 2 3 4 5	1 2 3 4 5	1 2 3 4 5	1 2 3 4 5	1 2 3 4 5
How good is the candidate's voice volume and voice speed?	1 2 3 4 5	1 2 3 4 5	1 2 3 4 5	1 2 3 4 5	1 2 3 4 5
How well does the candidate answer the questions?	1 2 3 4 5	1 2 3 4 5	1 2 3 4 5	1 2 3 4 5	1 2 3 4 5

Rating scale

1 = Needs a lot of work   2 = Needs some work   3 = Okay   4 = Good   5 = Excellent

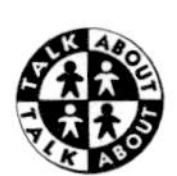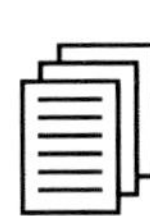

Activity 24 Interview – group rating scale

	Name:	Name:	Name:	Name:
Does the candidate answer any questions well in particular?				
What could the candidate improve about their answers?				
Does the candidate ask any questions at the end?				
Would you like to give any other feedback?				

Activity 24 Interview – individual rating scale

Name:		
Did you greet the interviewer appropriately?	Yes	No
How good is your eye contact?	1 2 3 4 5	
How good is your posture?	1 2 3 4 5	
How good is your ability to sit still?	1 2 3 4 5	
How good is your voice volume and speed?	1 2 3 4 5	
How well do you answer the questions?	1 2 3 4 5	
Did you answer any particular questions well?		
What could you improve about your answers?		
Did you ask any questions at the end?		
Do you have any other comments?		

Rating scale

1 = Needs a lot of work   2 = Needs some work   3 = Okay   4 = Good   5 = Excellent

---

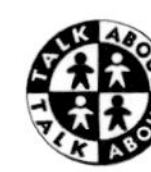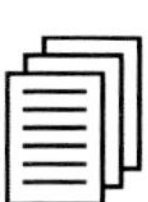

Activity 25 How do I look?

Preparation

Photocopy the worksheets. Cut out and laminate the clothing pictures. Cut out and laminate the appropriate/not appropriate headings and the individual clothing items.

This activity may take up to two sessions.

Instructions

- The group members take it in turns to turn over one of the pictures of the people in different clothes and think about how they look. Discuss the individual items (e.g. glasses, jeans, skirt, etc.) they are wearing and whether they are appropriate or inappropriate for an interview. How should someone look for an interview?

- You can also use the appropriate/not appropriate headings and sort the individual clothing pictures under these.

- The group can then fill in the worksheets with their answers. To make this activity easier, the group members can cut out the option words and stick them onto the individual worksheets.

- Look at the next series of pictures, involving body language – what is the difference between the examples. What is appropriate body language for an interview? The group can discuss what they think the rule is before the group leaders reveal the answers.

- If you feel that the group members need further work on these aspects of conversation skills, it is recommended that you consult the *Talkabout (2nd Edition)* book for additional activities.

Activity 25 How do I look?

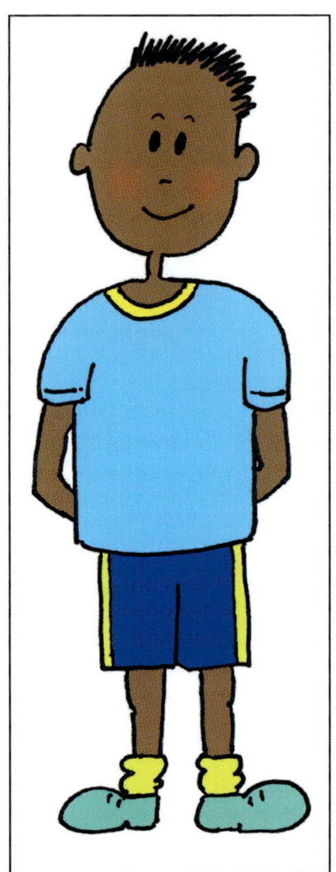 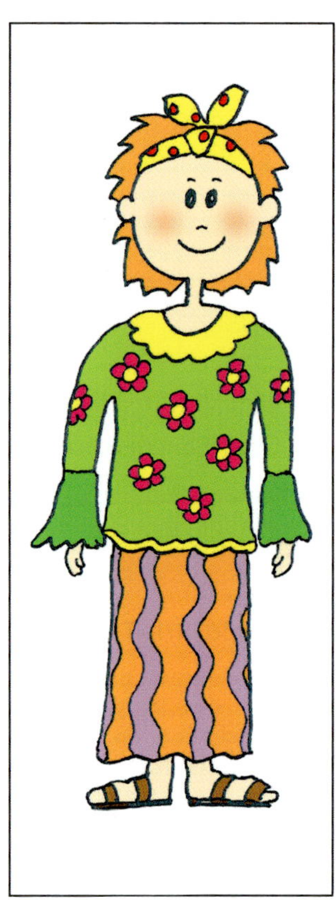 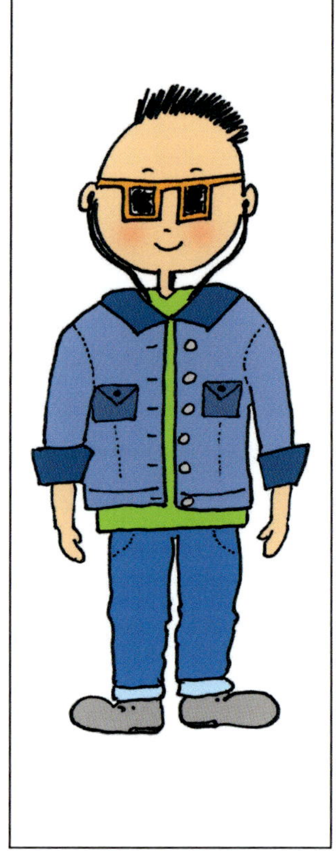 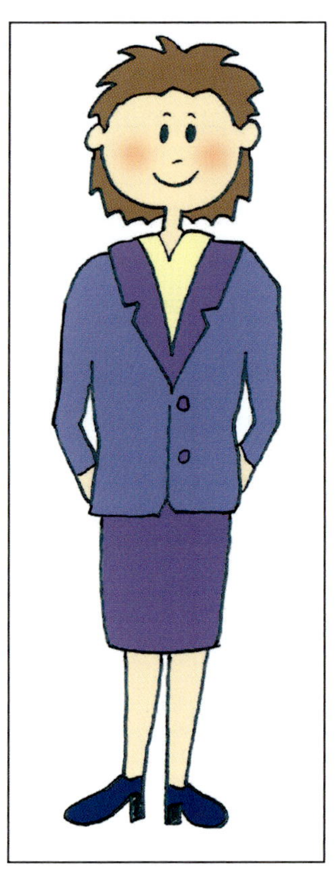

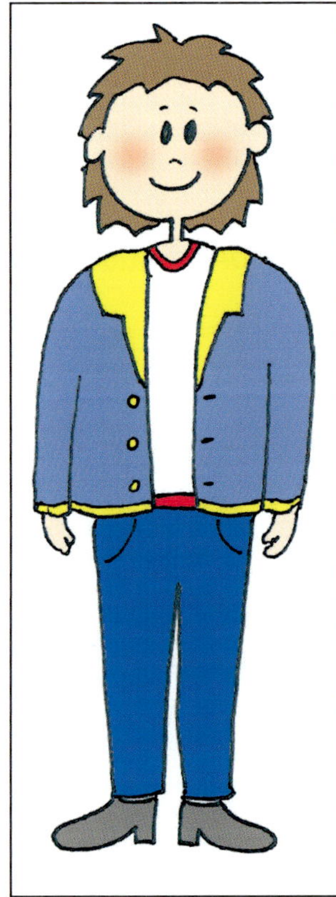 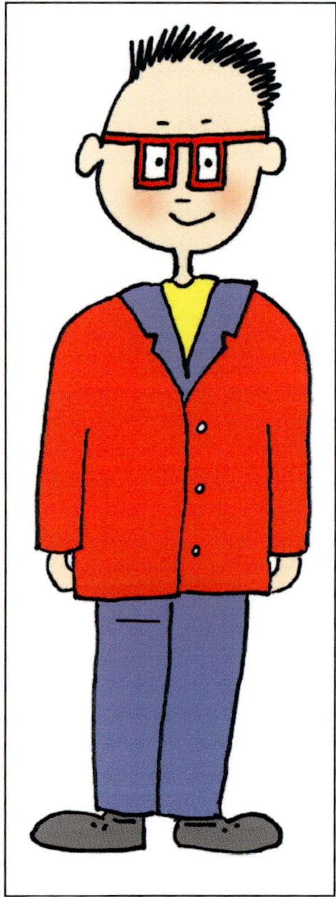 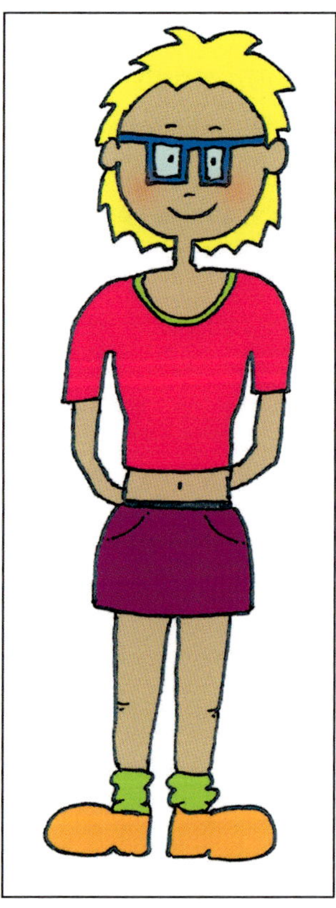 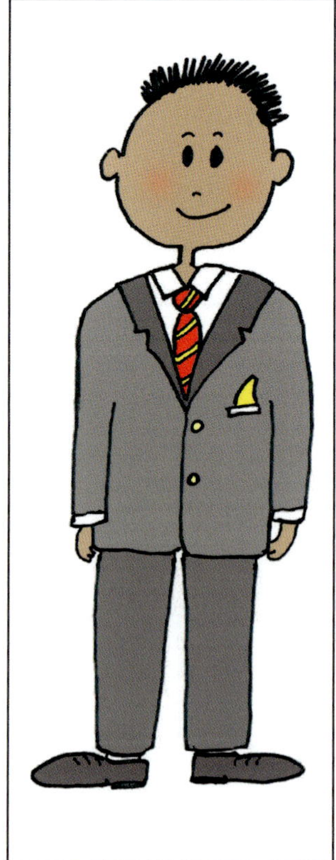

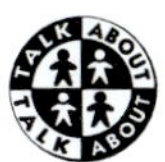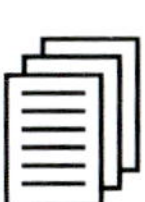

Activity 25 How do I look?

Write down or stick in six items that are appropriate to wear for interviews.

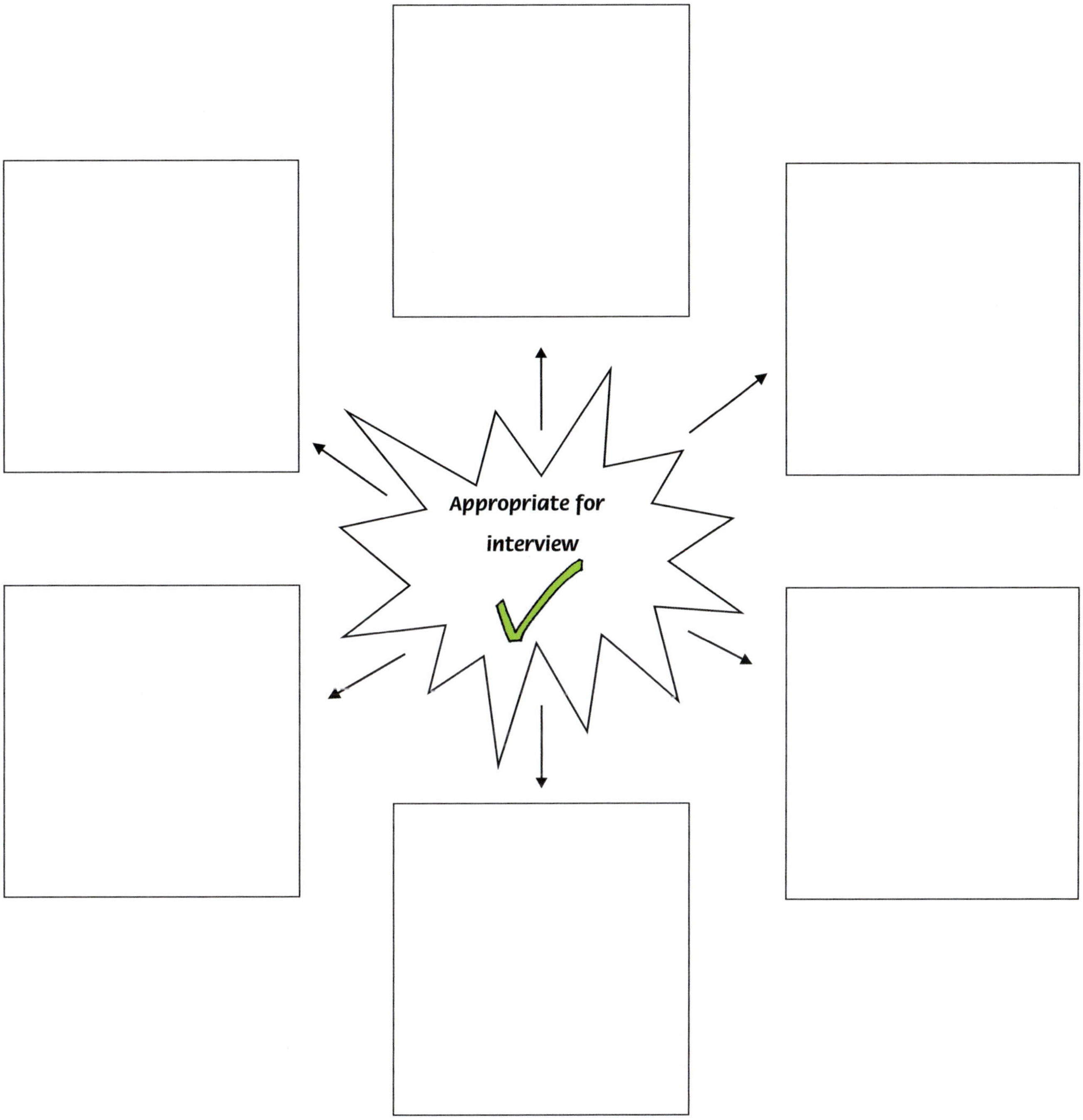

Activity 25 How do I look?

Write down or stick in six items that are not appropriate to wear for interviews.

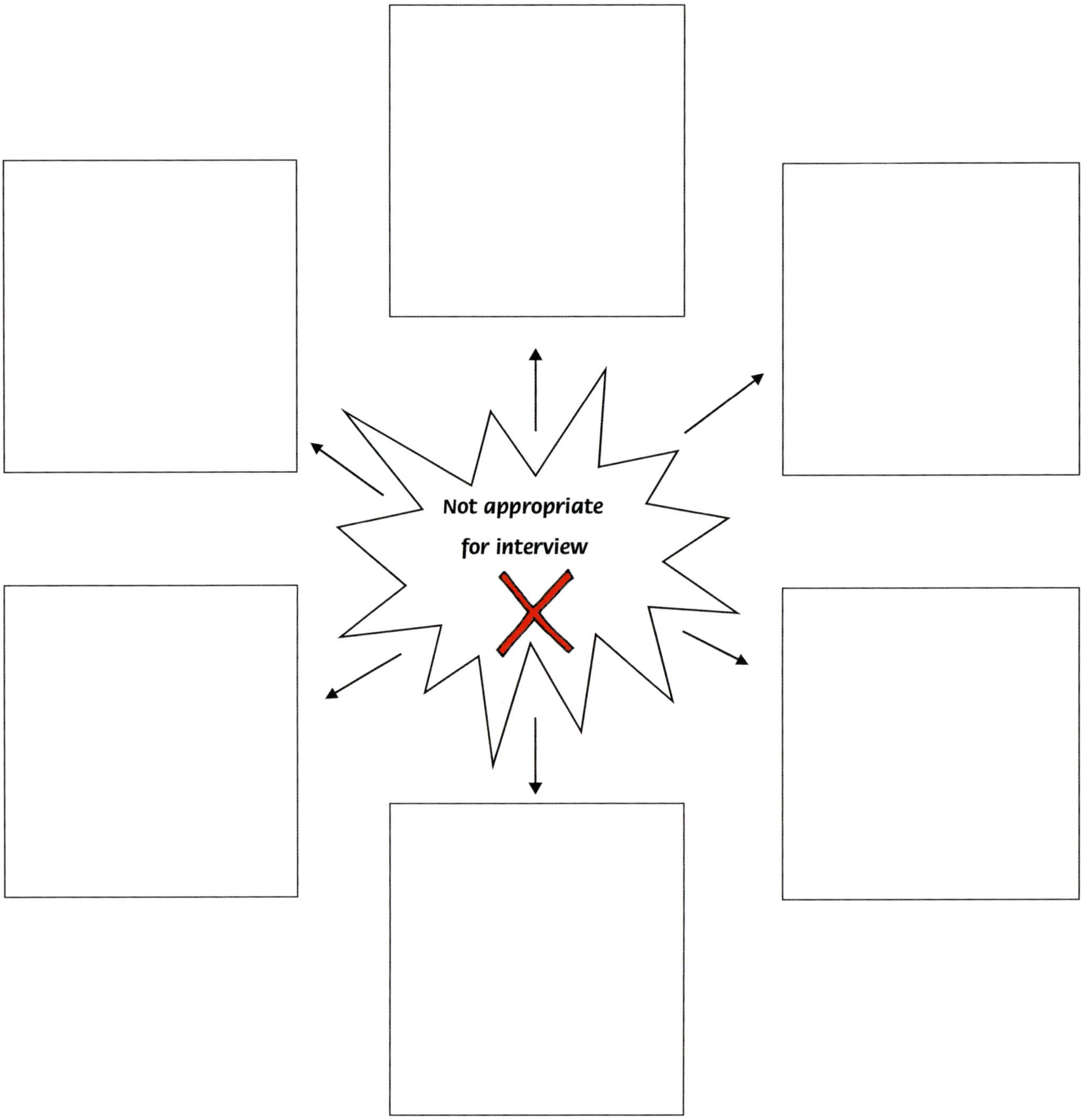

Not appropriate for interview

 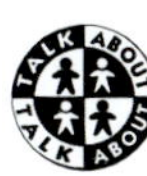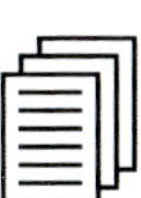

Activity 25 How do I look?

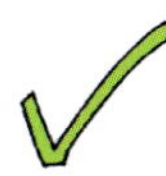	Appropriate

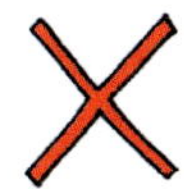	Not appropriate

Baseball cap	Colourful socks	Suit jacket
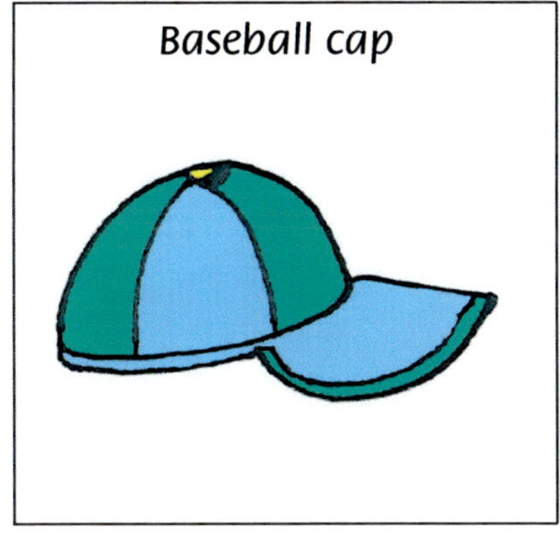	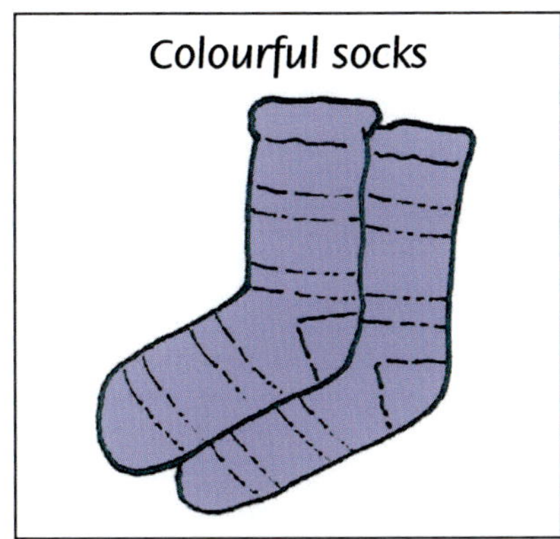	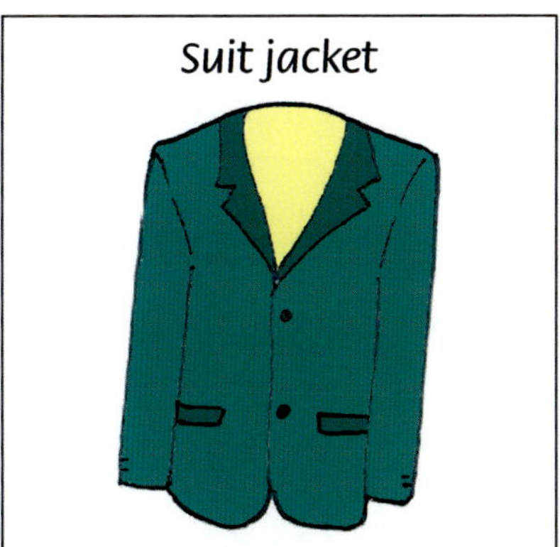
Bow tie	Miniskirt	Jeans
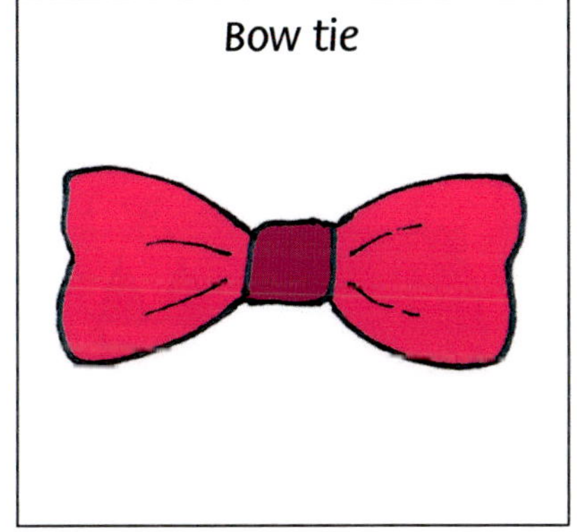	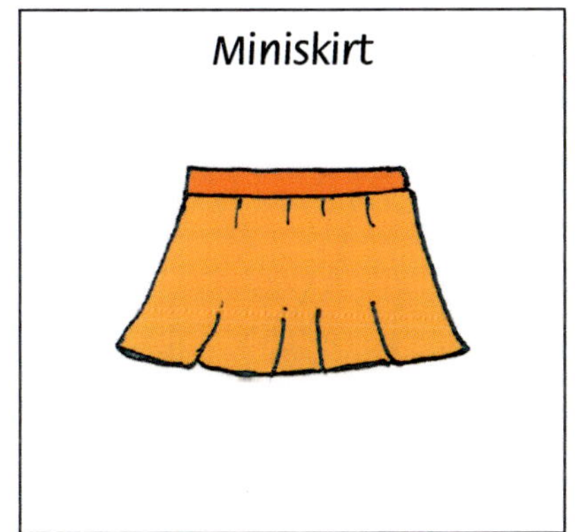	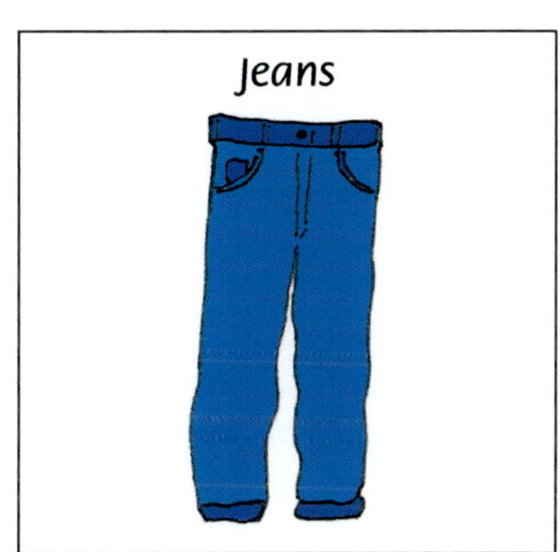
Tie	Stilettos	Smart shirt
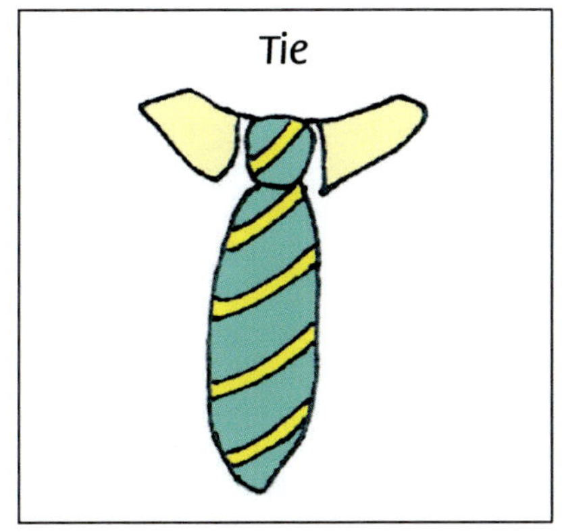	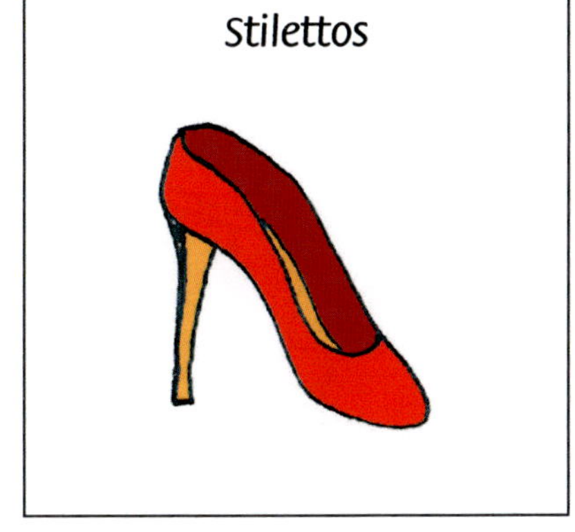	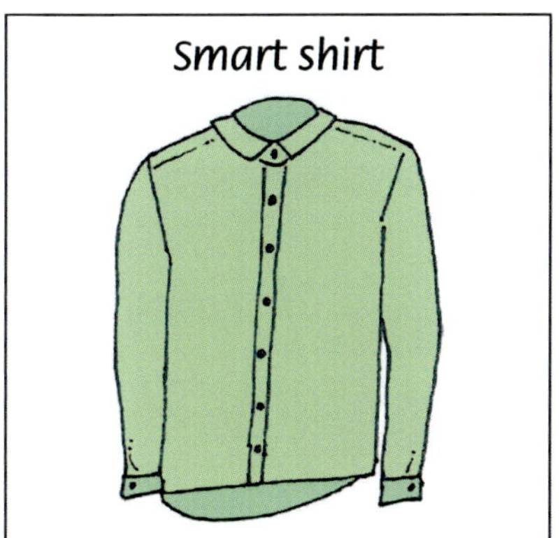

Activity 25 How do I look?

Small heeled shoes 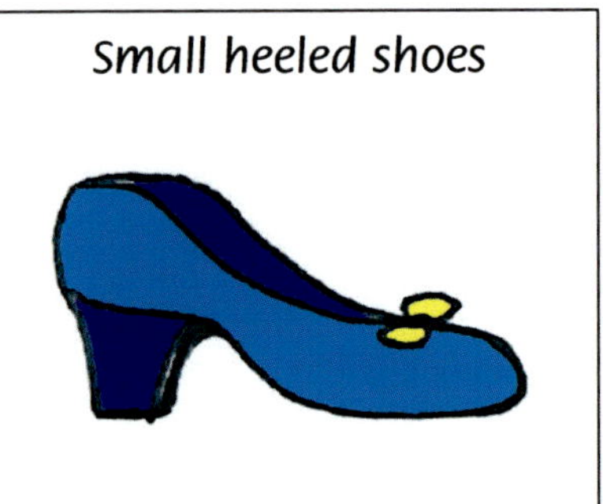	Black or brown shoes 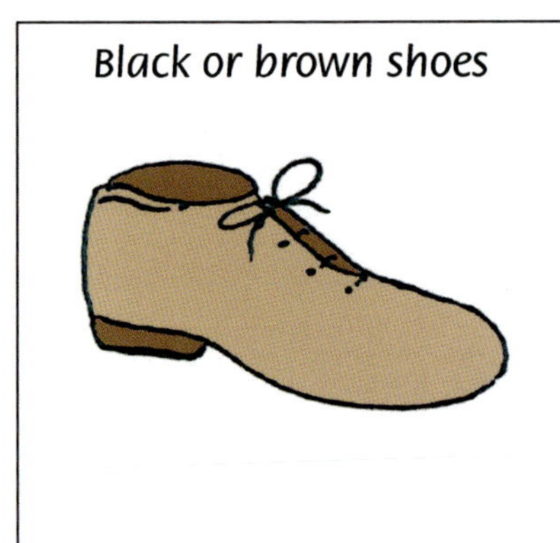	Sensible skirt 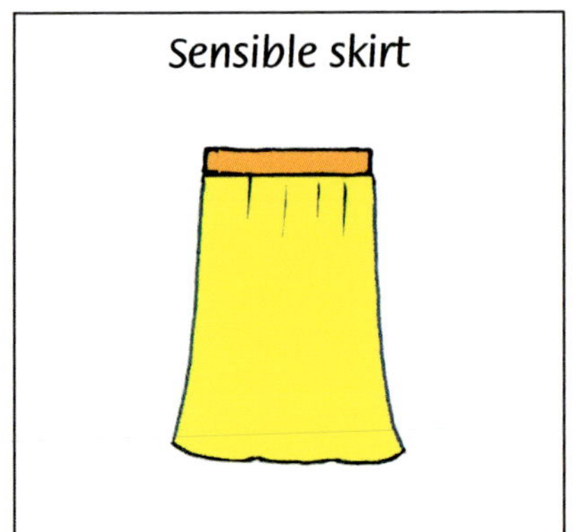
A watch 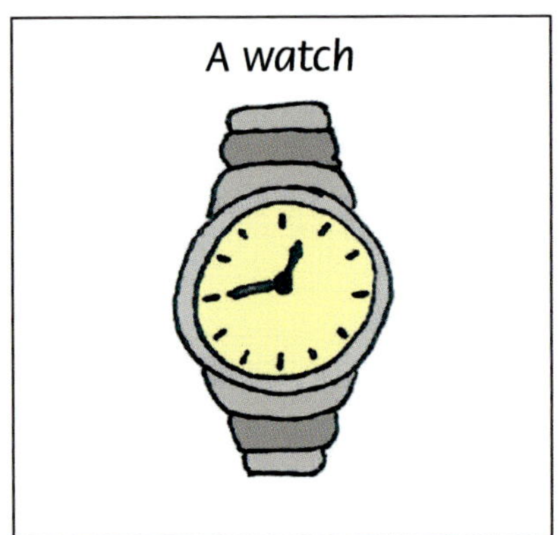	Suit trousers 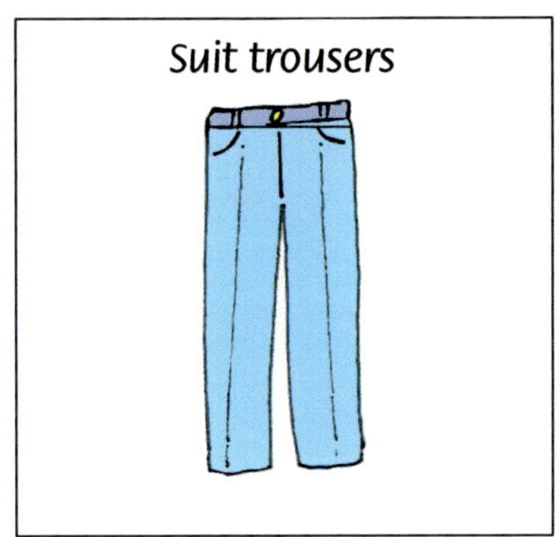	Trainers 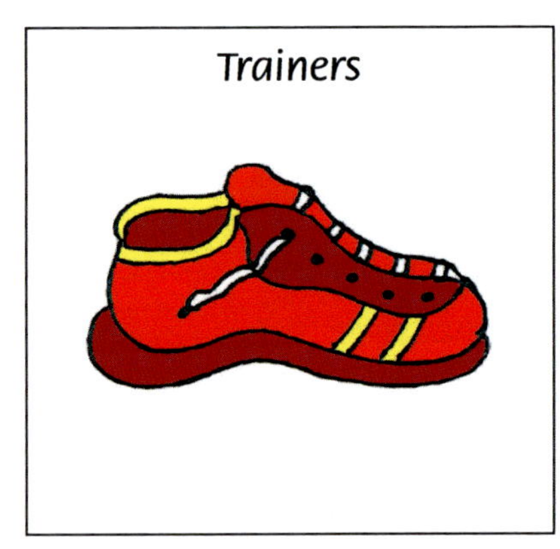
Glasses 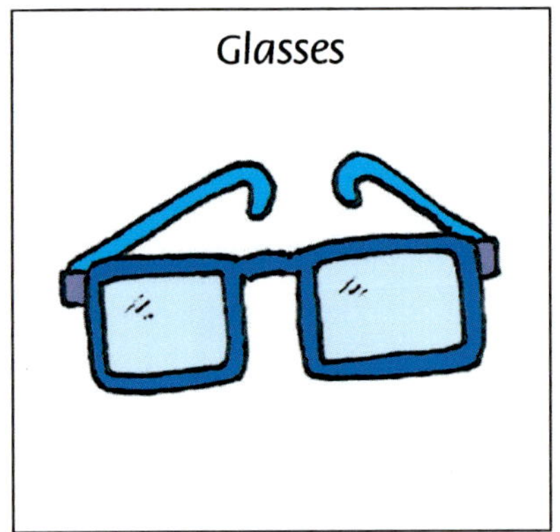	Blouse 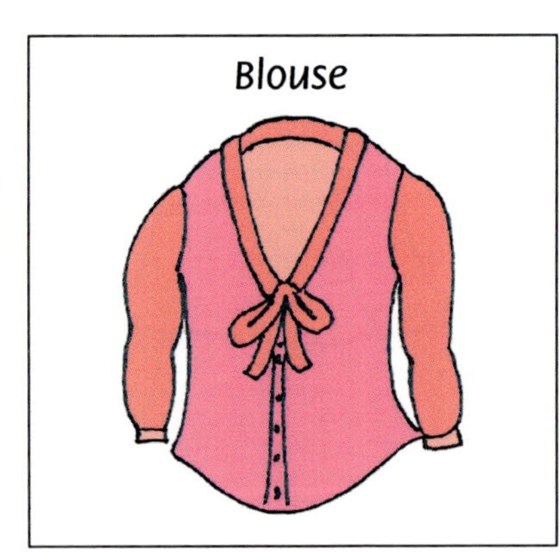	Swimming trunks or bikini 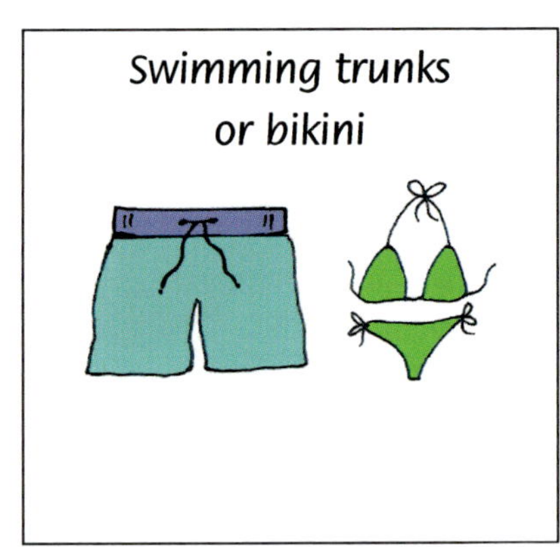
Flip flops 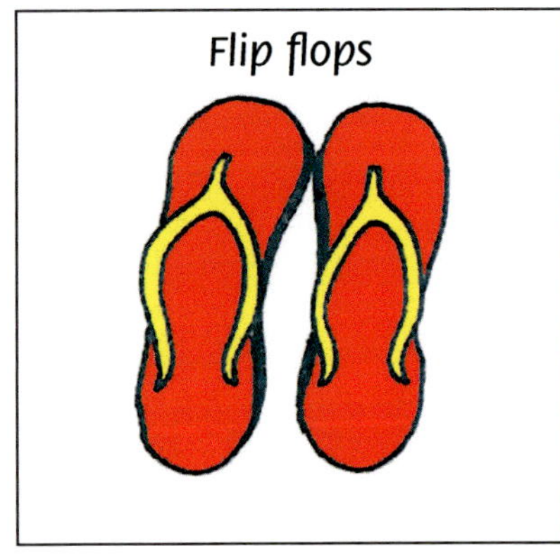	Lots of jewellery 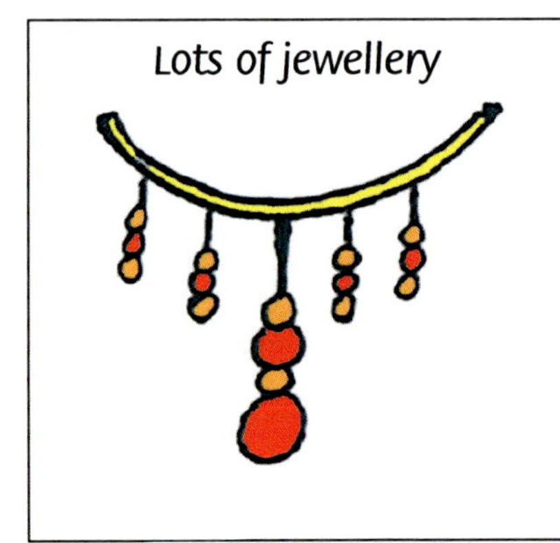	T-shirt 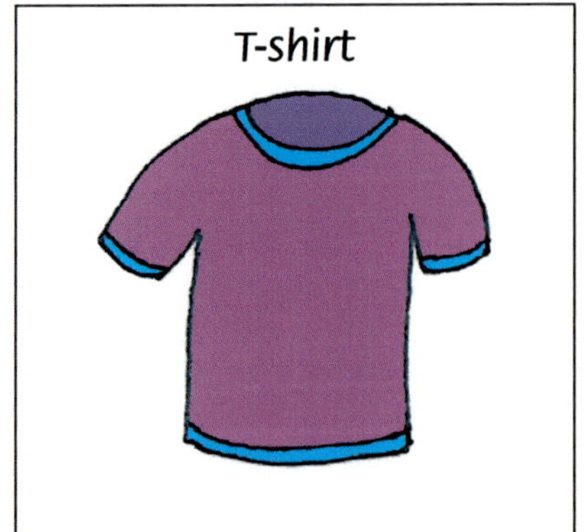

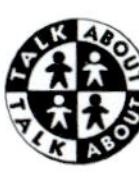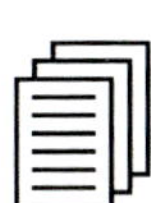

Activity 25 How do I look?

Eye contact

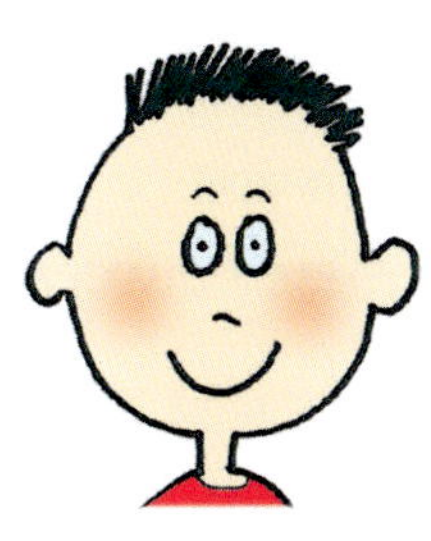

or

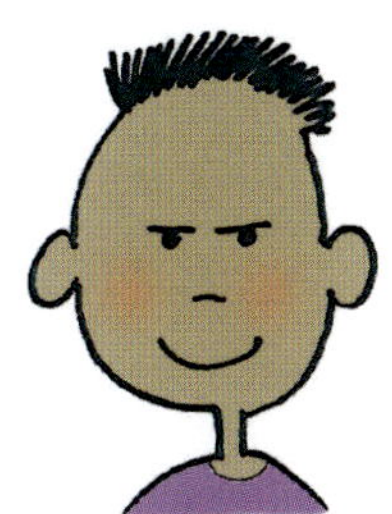

Facial expression

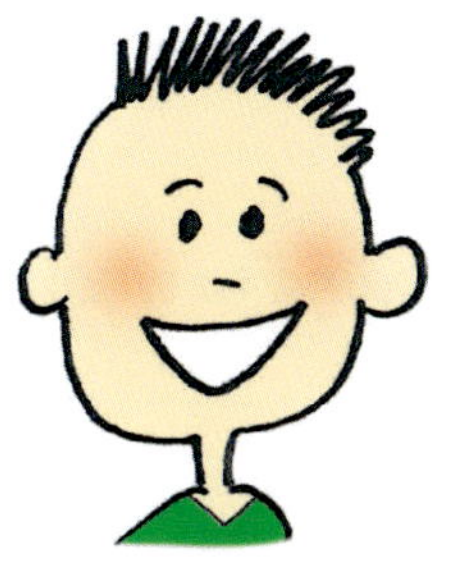

or

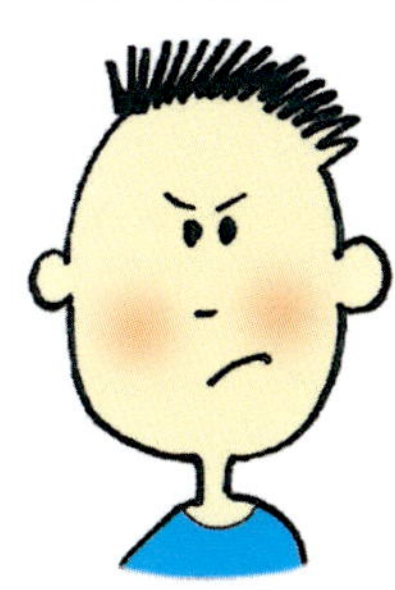

Distance

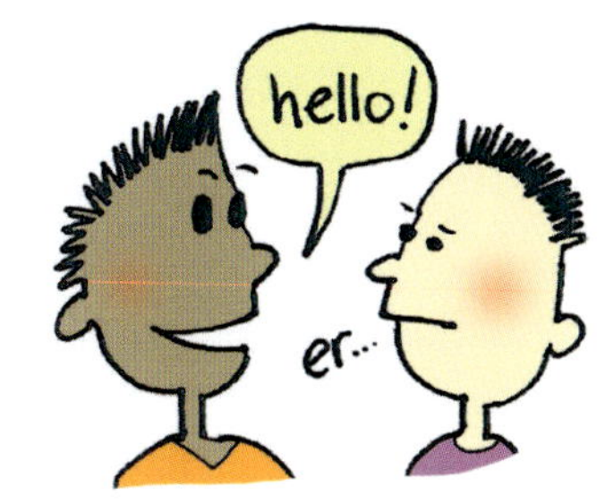

or

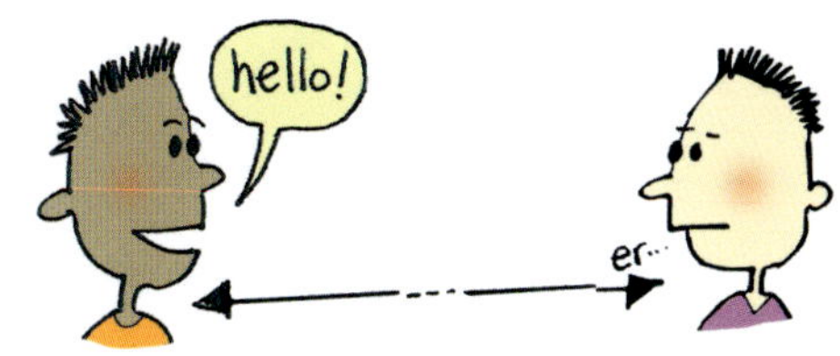

Touch

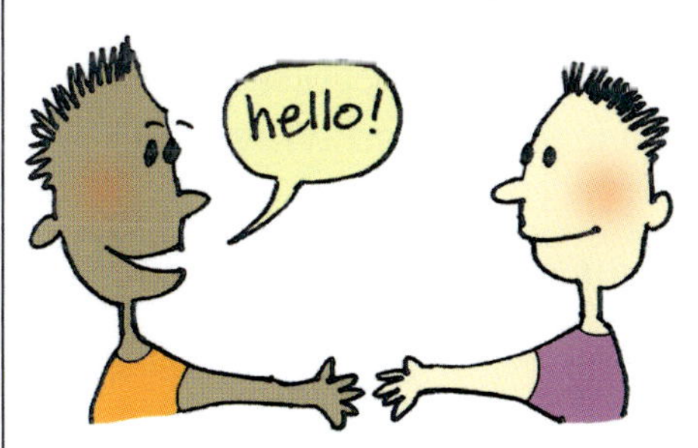

or

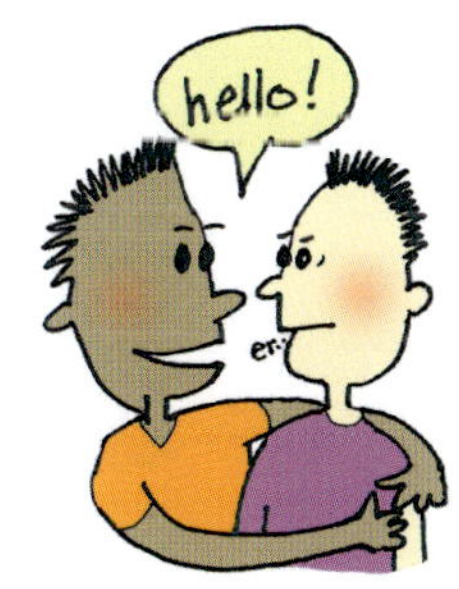

Posture

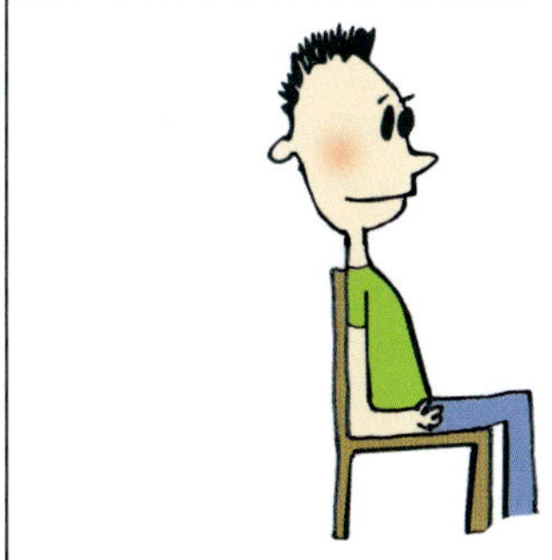

or

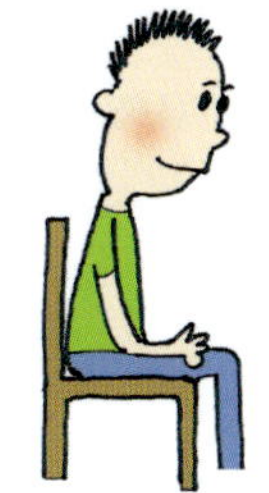

or

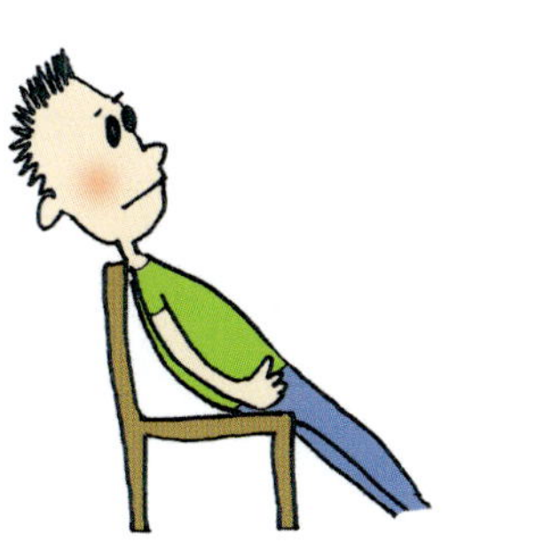

Activity 25 How do I look? Rules

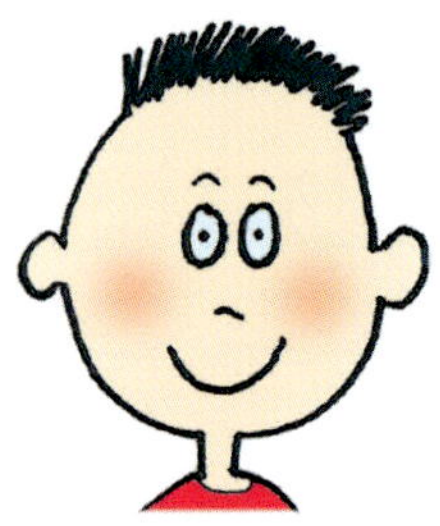

Eye contact
- Look towards the interviewer when they are talking to you.
- Looking at the person's eyes is great or look somewhere between their eyebrows and the tip of their nose.
- Look away for a few seconds sometimes. Try not to stare.

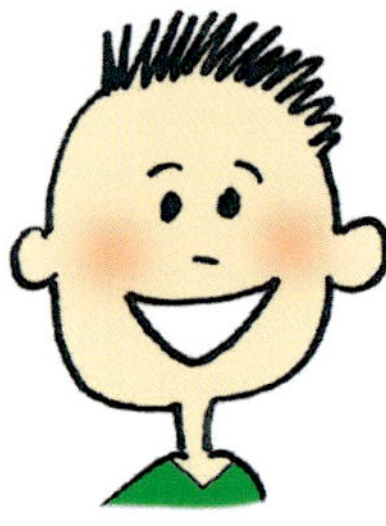

Facial expression
- Your face should match what you are saying.
- You should also make sure that your face is responding to what the interviewer is saying.
- Smiling helps you look friendly, confident and interested.

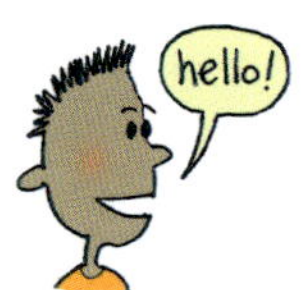
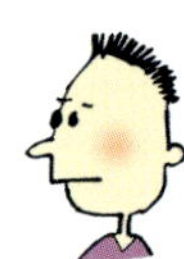

Distance
- Stand about one arm's length away from the person you are talking to.
- If you're taller than the person you're talking to or you don't know them very well, stand a bit further away.

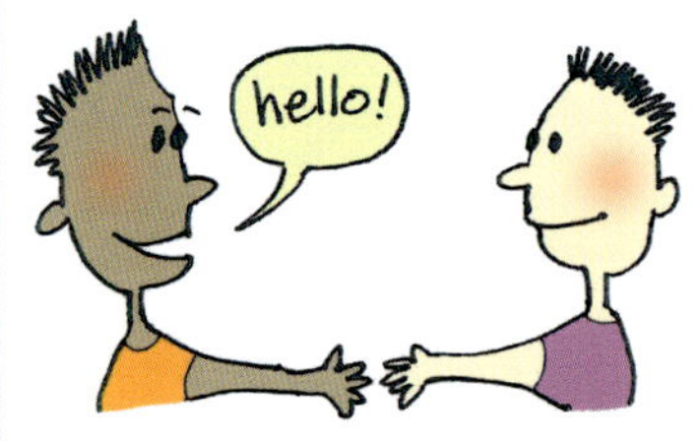

Touch
- It is important to shake the interviewer's hand when you greet them.
- Your handshake should be firm but not hard and should last around two to five seconds.

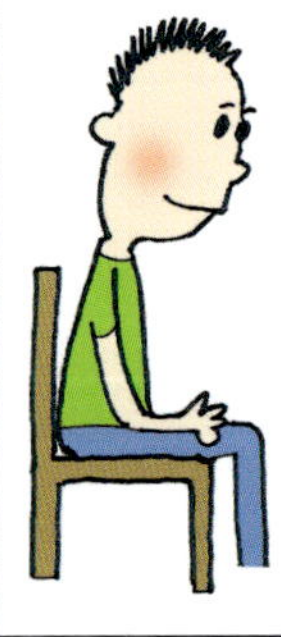

Posture
- Interviewers decide whether they like us within seven seconds of meeting us and this is partly based on posture.
- In an interview we should sit upright to show that we respect the interviewer and that we are listening.

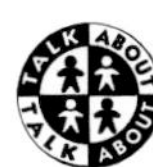

Activity 26 How do I sound?

Preparation

Each group leader will need a copy of the script. Photocopy the worksheet for each group member. This activity may take up to two sessions to complete.

Instructions

- Demonstrate an interview, following the script provided or improvising your own script (the questions are the same as the questions in Activity 24). In this demonstration, the group leader being interviewed will demonstrate poor listening, turn-taking, relevance, volume and rate in turn. (In the scripts, 'A' is the interviewer and 'B' is the interviewee.)

- Once the group leaders have finished each example, see if the group can identify the poor skills that the group leader is using. The group leaders should write the answers up on the board or flip chart. How does the group think that the group leaders can improve? Make sure they cover all the relevant rules written in the group leaders' rules sheet.

- Provide the students with the work sheets and support them to fill in the rules with the correct information.

- If you feel that the group members need further work on these aspects of conversation skills, it is recommended that you consult the *Talkabout (2nd Edition)* book for additional activities.

Activity 26 How do I sound?

Listening:

A: Hi, how are you?

B: (Looking around the room, leaning back in chair)

A: Okay… Well, we'll get started with the interview. What can you tell me about yourself or your personality?

B: (Looking around, fidgeting with a pen, frowning) Huh?

A: Uh, the question is: what can you tell me about yourself or your personality?

B: (Still not looking at A, looking unimpressed, checking phone) Sorry, what?

A: (Exasperated) I said, what can you tell me about yourself or your personality?

B: (Frowning) Oh, right. You need to speak up a bit. I'm very hard-working, I'm very friendly and I have great listening skills.

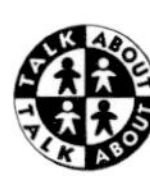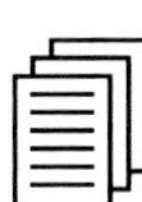

Activity 26 How do I sound?

Turn-taking:

A: Hi, how are you?

B: I'm alright, thank you.

A: (At the same time) Excellent, well, we'll start with the interview.

B: (At the same time) It's great to have this opportunity.

A: Right. What can you tell me about yourself or your personality?

B: (Before he's finished speaking) I'm very hard-working, very friendly and I have great listening skills. I've developed these over the course of an extensive career in computing. I can tell you I'm hard-working because I focus on what I need to do and when I need to do it. I'm friendly – I'm able to build up relationships very quickly and often become really great friends with the people that I work with. And… what was the last one? (A looks bored and sighs) Oh yes, I have great listening skills, I'm able to lend an ear to someone if they need some help and really enjoy answering people's questions. (Pause, while seeming to think, looking away)

A: (At the same time) Great answer, we'll move on to the next question.

B: (At the same time) And I just really enjoy working with people, I'm really passionate about that.

Activity 26 How do I sound?

Relevance:

A: Hi, how are you?

B: I'm great, thank you. I had a brilliant breakfast on the way here in a little restaurant, eggs and bacon with toast and then a really nice cup of coffee to round things off.

A: Right, well, shall we start with the interview.

B: Yes. I haven't had a breakfast like that for ages, the eggs were poached and I think they must have fried the bacon.

A: Okay, sounds like a great breakfast. What can you tell me about yourself or your personality?

B: Well, I'm very hard-working, I'm very friendly and I have great listening skills. I'm also really hungry still, do you know anywhere nearby that I could get some more eggs and bacon? In fact, can I get a cup of coffee here?

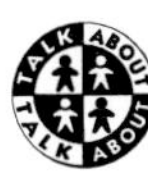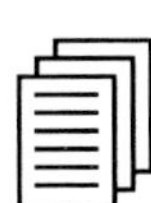

Activity 26 How do I sound?

Volume (1):

A: Hi, how are you?

B: (Very loud) I'm great, thank you!

A: Right, well, we'll get started with the interview.

B: (Very loud) Excellent!

A: So, what can you tell me about yourself or your personality?

B: (Very loud) I'm very hard-working, I'm very friendly and I have great listening skills.

Volume (2):

A: Hi, how are you?

B: (Mumbling) I'm alright, how are you?

A: Pardon?

B: (A little bit louder) I'm alright, how are you?

A: Oh, I'm good, thank you. Shall we start with the interview? What can you tell me about yourself or your personality?

B: (Mumbling again) Oh, I'm really friendly, I'm hard-working and I have great listening skills. I think.

Activity 26 How do I sound?

Rate (1):

A: Hi, how are you?

B: (Very quickly) I'm great, thanks, how are you?

A: Good, thank you. We'll start the interview then, what can you tell me about yourself or your personality?

B: (Very quickly again) Oh, I have lots of skills and abilities and hobbies, I have great listening skills and I'm hard-working, friendly, good fun to be around, great sense of humour. I like going climbing and going to restaurants.

Rate (2):

A: Hi, how are you?

B: (Very slowly) Oh, I'm great. Thanks. How are you?

A: I'm fine, shall we start? What can you tell me about yourself or your personality?

B: (Very slowly) I'm really friendly. And hard-working. And I've got a great sense of humour.

Activity 26 How do I sound? Rules

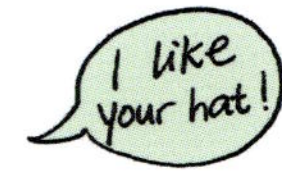

1. Use good eye contact.
2. Use appropriate facial expressions – look interested in their questions.
3. Use an open posture or lean forward.
4. Avoid fidgeting with objects.
5. Turn our phone off.

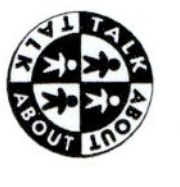

1. Talk about topics that are appropriate to the interview.
2. Listen to the interviewer and answer their questions specifically.

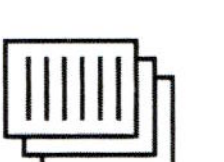

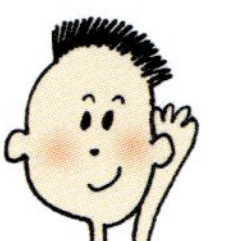

1. Keep quiet and let the interviewer ask the questions.
2. Take time over our answers, but don't speak for a very long time.
3. We can use eye contact to let the interviewer know we've finished.

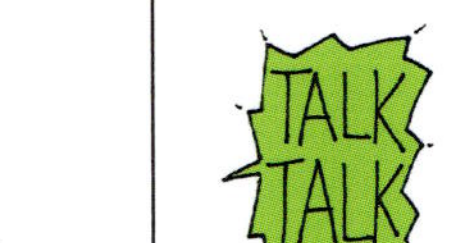

1. Use an appropriate volume – not too loud and not too quiet.
2. Use an appropriate rate of speech – not to slow and not too quick.
3. Remember to speak clearly and not mumble.

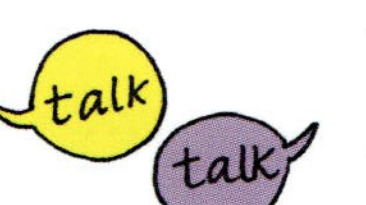

Activity 26 How do I sound? Rules

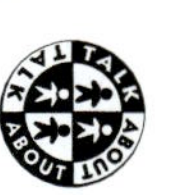

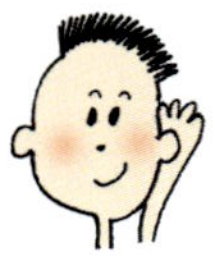

To show we are listening in an interview, we should:

1. ....
2. ....
3. ....
4. ....
5. ....

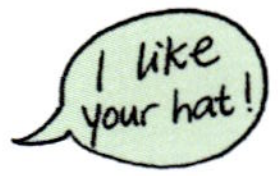

To show we are being relevant in an interview, we should:

1. ....
   ....
2. ....
   ....

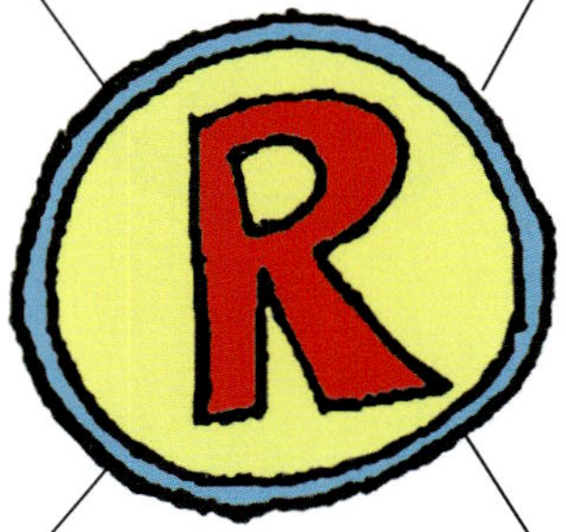

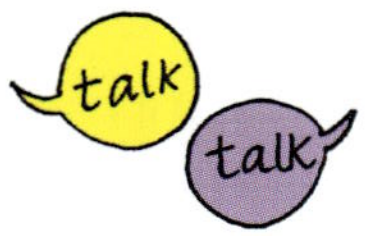

To show good turn-taking in an interview, we should:

1. ....
   ....
2. ....
   ....
3. ....
   ....

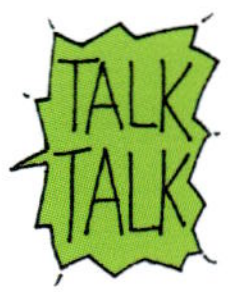

To talk well in an interview, we should:

1. ....
   ....
2. ....
   ....
3. ....
   ....

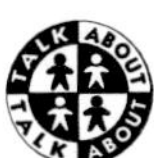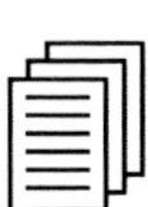

Activity 27 Good and bad answers

Preparation

Photocopy one script for each group leader. The group members should have a copy of the questions from Activity 24.

Instructions

- Similar to the last activity, demonstrate two interview situations, the first having poor answers to the interview questions and the second having good answers. Both group leaders should keep their body language and the way they talk appropriate so that this does not distract from the answers.

- If you feel confident, the group members can take one of the other job descriptions and improvise their own good and bad interviews.

- After each bad answer, discuss what was bad about the answer and what the person could do to make it better. What do they need to mention in the content of their answer? For example, mentioning money in the answer to 'Why do you want to work here?' is frowned upon, but mentioning that the person is ambitious and they'd like opportunities for progression is a positive spin on this.

- Once the group leaders have finished the bad answers, see if the group can think of the rules for answering the questions. What do you need to do to answer the questions well? Provide the students with the worksheet and ask them to write these rules down or alternatively, just discuss them in a group.

- Go through the scripts for the good answers. After every question, discuss with the group what the good answer had in it. They can then write this down on the worksheet.

Activity 27 Good and bad answers

Job:

Office worker: Use a computer to maintain files and records. Answer the phone. Do basic finance tasks, like issue invoices. Sort incoming and outgoing mail. Make sure there's enough stationery in the office.

Bad answers:

A: What can you tell me about yourself or your personality?

B: Well, that's a big question! Where do I start? I was born in London, 1986. I grew up in the country outside it though. I went to a small school and was quite clever and had loads of friends. I moved up to secondary school and didn't really enjoy lessons, but me and my friends went out a lot. I've lost contact with most of them now. Anyway, when I left school I started skateboarding and now I really enjoy doing that when I'm not working. I'm a really great person and I think that if you just hired me then you'd get to know me.

A: Can you tell me your three biggest strengths?

B: One of my strengths is that I'm awesome, so good at all the work that I do. I'm pretty sure I learn quickly as well and sometimes I'm friendly, but not in the morning when I've just woken up and not had a cup of coffee yet. No one talk to me then! That's three, isn't it?

A: Can you tell me one weakness about yourself?

B: Hmm, I'm not sure there is one to be honest. I'm perfect in every way and I'm pretty sure you'll see that when you hire me. I guess if I had to choose one, it's that sometimes I get annoyed when people aren't as good as me at their jobs, but that's their fault really, they should be better at their job.

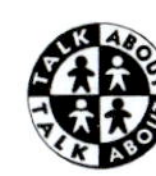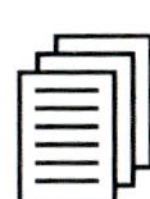

Activity 27 Good and bad answers

A: Why do you want to work here?

B: Well, for starters, I really need the money and this place is only around the corner from my house, so it won't take me long to get here in the morning.

A: What experience or skills do you have that might help you do this job?

B: Well, I'm amazing at video games so I'm really good at using a mouse or a tablet or something like that. I'm quite funny and that might help you out with the other people in the office, you know, get them pepped up! I'm also a really quick worker so I can get something done and then I can go home for the rest of the day, right?

A: What do you enjoy doing in your spare time?

B: I know I already said this, but I love skateboarding and playing computer games. They're difficult, but you can chill out at the same time. They're much more fun than working, I can never wait to get to the end of the day so I can go home and skate!

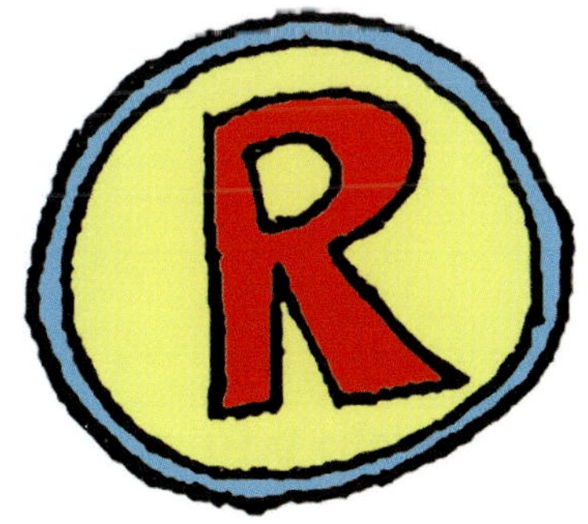

Rules to cover in discussion:

To answer questions well, we should:

- Keep all our answers relevant to the job role as much as possible

- Make sure to listen to the interviewer's question

- When we are asked an open question, give as much detail as necessary but be careful not to give too much

Activity 27 Good and bad answers

Good answers:

A: What can you tell me about yourself or your personality?

B: I've always had an interest in computers and have grown up using them. I've just finished my college course in Information Technology, including a module on coding and programming, and really enjoyed learning things that I didn't know about how computers work.

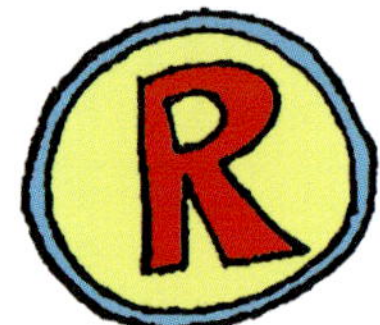

Rule: Talk about your interests and experiences in education and at home and how these are relevant to the job you are interviewing for.

A: Can you tell me your three biggest strengths?

B: I'm very organised and use my calendar on my phone and computer to keep me on track with projects and deadlines. I'm determined and won't put a project away without giving my best go at it. I'm also very friendly and get on with people well so I find it easy to fit into teams.

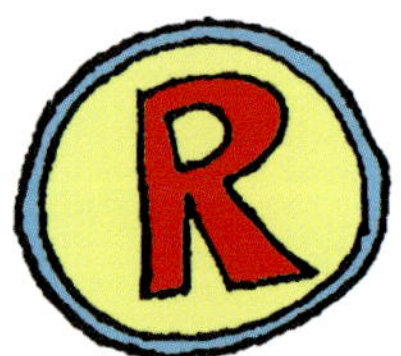

Rule: Prepare for this by thinking of three strengths. Develop this by explaining how they would help you do the job you want to do.

Activity 27 Good and bad answers

A: Can you tell me one weakness about yourself?

B: Sometimes I'm a bit too enthusiastic during my work, which means that I'll say yes to jobs that I don't have time to do. I have started to identify these moments though and will say no if I don't have time, or I'll seek help from one of my colleagues.

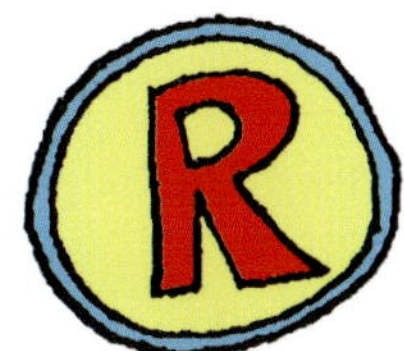

Rule: Prepare for this question by coming up with something that is more difficult for you. Think about what you can do to fix it or what you are already doing to help change the difficulty.

A: Why do you want to work here?

B: As I've only just qualified from college, I'm looking to start putting all the aspects of my learning into practice in a business environment alongside a like-minded team. Your company has a great reputation for developing people's skills and the projects that you've worked on previously look incredibly interesting and motivating.

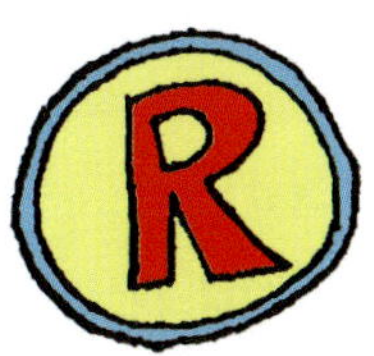

Rule: The answer to this question will involve doing some research on the company you are interviewing for and knowing what they create or do. Once you know this, you can talk about how much you will like doing the job you've applied for.

Activity 27 Good and bad answers

A: What experience or skills do you have that might help you do this job?

B: I did my work experience in an office environment and learnt a lot about the different systems they used and how to communicate with people who want to use those systems. I'm very creative so I'm able to think about how to do things differently that might be better for the company and I'm able to do this independently. I'm also very good at listening to people's difficulties with computers and will be able to help.

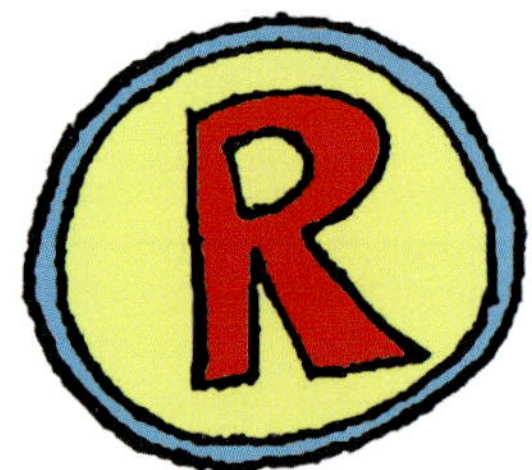

Rule: Choose three skills that will be useful for the job you want to do and explore these individually. They might be related to a time at school, college or another job.

A: What do you enjoy doing in your spare time?

B: I like to develop my computer skills in different ways, practising website creation and coding. I also play guitar and practise this in a band and I think this helps me with my creativity.

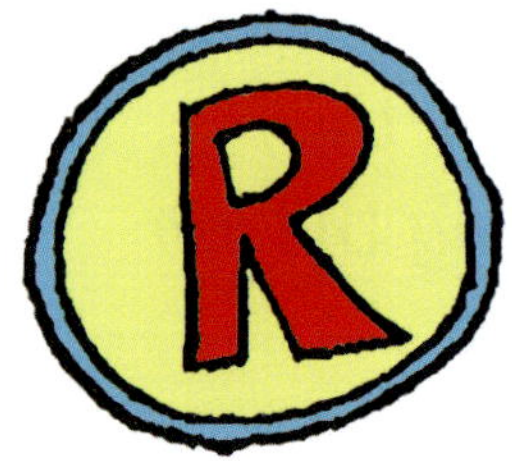

Rule: Explain what your hobbies are and how can these help you with the job? These might show you're learning outside of school or work.

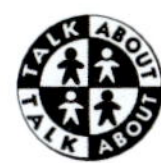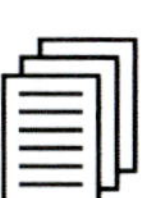

Activity 27 Good and bad answers

What are the rules for answering questions?

1. ....

2. ....

3. ....

What are the rules for the individual questions?

1. What can you tell me about yourself or your personality?

> Rule: ....
>
> ....

2. Can you tell me your three biggest strengths?

> Rule: ....
>
> ....

3. Can you tell me one weakness about yourself?

> Rule: ....
>
> ....

4. Why do you want to work here?

> Rule: ....
>
> ....

5. What experience or skills do you have that might help you do this job?

> Rule: ....
>
> ....

6. What do you enjoy doing in your spare time?

> Rule: ....
>
> ....

Activity 28 Interview questions

Preparation

Photocopy the worksheet.

Instructions

- Remind the group members of the topics covered in the last session. Explain that today they will be writing their answers to the interview questions.

- Provide each group member with a copy of the worksheet as well as the job descriptions from Activity 24. The group members should choose a job to apply for and the group leaders can support them to go through the questions, filling in an answer for each one. To help with this the group members can use their previous answers to their strengths, weakness, interests and skills, e.g. their advert or CV.

- This can also take place as a discussion in pairs. The group members could go through the list of questions and identify what they would like to say for each one.

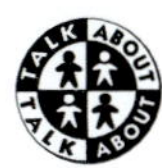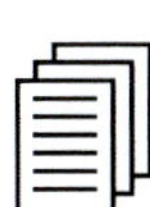

Activity 28 Interview questions

1. What can you tell me about yourself or your personality?

What interests do you have?

....

What were your favourite lessons at school or college?

....

How are these related to the job you've chosen to apply for?

....

....

....

2. Can you tell me your three biggest strengths?

Quality 1: ....

How could this help you in the chosen job?

....

....

Quality 2: ....

How could this help you in the chosen job?

....

....

Quality 3: ....

How could this help you in the chosen job?

....

....

Activity 28 Interview questions

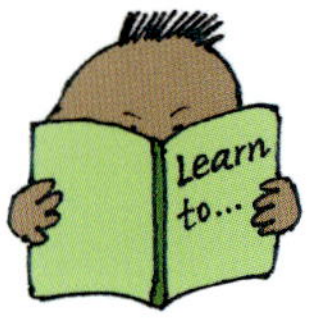

3. Can you tell me one weakness about yourself?

One thing you could work on: ....

What have you done to make it better already?

....

....

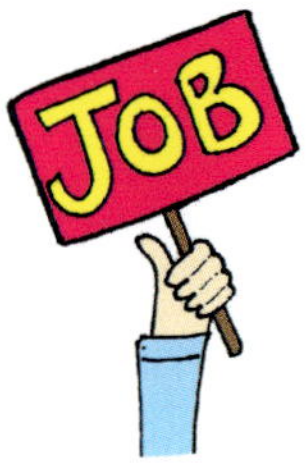

4. Why do you want to work here?

What do you like about the job you have chosen?

....

....

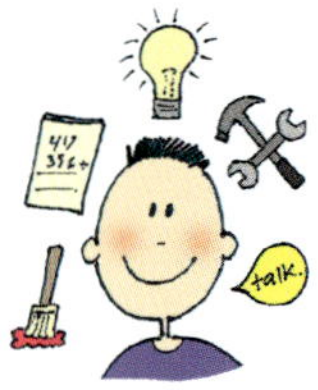

5. What experience or skills do you have that might help you do this job?

Have you done any similar work experience to your chosen job? What was it and why could it help you?

....

....

What skills do you have that could help?

Skill 1: ....

Skill 2: ....

Skill 3: ....

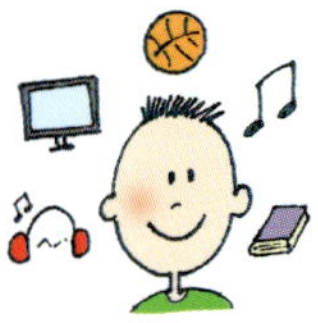

6. What do you enjoy doing in your spare time?

What are your hobbies?

....

How could they help you with the job?

....

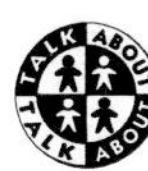
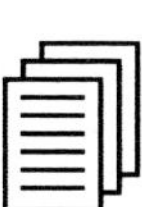

Activity 29 Second interview

Preparation

Use the same job descriptions and interview questions as the first interview at the beginning of this topic. The group members will also need their work from Activity 28.

Instructions

- Provide the group members with their work from the last session so that they have an opportunity to look at their answers.

- Run the interviews in the same way as the first interviews so that an accurate comparison can be made. The students should either work as a pair or take it in turns to leave and carry out their interview with a group leader. Meanwhile, the other group leader should carry out a group cohesion activity to ensure that group members do not feel too much anxiety.

Activity 30 Comparing interviews

Preparation

Photocopy the evaluation forms from Activity 24.

Instructions

- If the group leaders recorded the interviews from the last session and the students feel confident enough, you can watch these back as a group. If not, the group members can watch them individually and score themselves.

- If they watch the videos, they should use the evaluation forms to score themselves and the others. Any group criticism should be constructive and include possible improvements. Encourage compliments, asking each member for one good thing that a group member has done in the interview.

- Provide the students with the original forms and compare the results. Have they improved their scores? Are there things they still need to work on?

- Keep these scores as evidence of progress.

Topic 5 – Workplace relationships

Objectives

To understand who to talk to in certain situations at work.

To understand what is and isn't appropriate for small talk and develop conversation starters.

To become aware of different strategies that will help deal with conflict.

To develop teamworking skills.

To complete the programme and reflect on any progress made.

Timing

This topic will take up to five sessions to complete.

Activity	Description
Introducing workplace relationships (Activity 31)	The group members take turns to decide who would be the most appropriate person at work to talk to about different situations.
Small talk (Activity 32)	The group members decide on what topics are appropriate and inappropriate for small talk and then think of some conversation starters and follow-up questions.
Dealing with conflict (Activity 33)	The group members take turns to read out a scenario and discuss how to solve the conflict. They then complete a worksheet detailing positive approaches to conflict in the workplace.
Stranded (Activity 34)	The group carry out a team-building exercise designed to work on important skills needed to work in a team successfully.
It's a wrap! (Activity 35)	The group members celebrate their work over the year and think about what they've learnt and achieved. This is designed to be the final activity in the programme. If you are planning to carry out activities from Topic 6, do this activity once you have finished those.

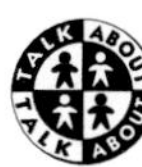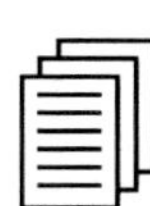

Activity 31 Introducing workplace relationships

Preparation

Photocopy, cut out and laminate the job titles and stick them on different pieces of paper or write the job titles on a flip chart or whiteboard in columns. Photocopy and cut out the workplace scenarios.

Instructions

- Let the group members know that when we start work somewhere new, we are thrown into a workplace with lots of different people. Some of these people might have been working there for a long time and some might be new. They will be of different ages, races, cultures, sexualities and religions, and everyone will have different personalities and ways of working.

- Define each of the job titles and ensure the group understand the meaning of each one. They may need to do research before beginning this activity if they are unsure what the job titles mean.

- Once they understand the definitions of each, the group members can go through the scenarios from the worksheet, taking turns to pick a card. Who would they discuss the problem with? Who would they do the activity with? For example, would you go for a coffee after work with your boss? Write each scenario under the appropriate job title. Discuss the concept of formal/informal relationships.

- See if the group members can apply these job titles to the setting that they are in, for example, if the group takes place in the school, who is the manager? Who are colleagues? Who are the customers?

- Reflect on the answers the group members have given. Are there any that they might feel uncomfortable with? Or any that they feel would be appropriate for another member of staff? Can they come up with any other scenarios?

Activity 31 Introducing workplace relationships

Manager

Colleague

Administrator

Supervisor

Friend at work

Customers

Another company's staff

Company director

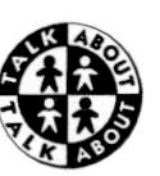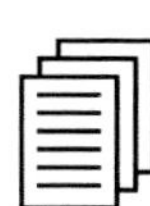

Activity 31 Introducing workplace relationships

You want to go into town after work for a coffee	You need to report an incidence of bullying
You've burnt yourself and need some first aid	You need help with a project
You want to complain about another member of staff	You need to introduce yourself professionally
You chat about your weekend and ask about another person's	You need some time off for a dentist appointment
You don't like part of your job	You want a pay rise
You offer to make a cup of tea	You know a way that the company could improve
You need to tell someone that you're not very well	You disagree with something in someone else's project
You go for a cigarette break	You need to organise a training course for your project
You need to dress professionally to meet them	You want to say that someone's done a good job
You want advice about a relationship outside work	You'd like to go on a date with someone at work
You have small talk with someone	You're angry at someone because they do something wrong

Activity 32 Small talk

Preparation

Photocopy, cut out and laminate the topic cards and print out the appropriate/not appropriate worksheet on A3 paper or photocopy the cards on A4 paper for each group member.

Instructions

- Discuss the benefits of developing positive workplace relationships with the group. Why do they think that it's a good thing to have positive relationships at work? Make sure to cover the fact that it increases job satisfaction, productivity, health and overall quality of life.

- Ask the group members to define small talk – what do they think it is? The definition is: polite conversation about unimportant topics that happen socially. Discuss its importance in creating initial relationships when starting a job. Small talk is useful for developing relationships and starting conversations when we don't know what else to say.

- Go through the pile of cards and take it in turns to decide whether a topic is appropriate or not appropriate for small talk. Once all the cards have been used, see if the group can name any more topics that would be good for small talk. If the group would work better individually, then provide each group member with the appropriate/not appropriate worksheets and ask them to cut out the individual topics and stick them onto the correct sheet.

- After this, the group can use the 'Questions' worksheet and either work individually or in pairs to come up with ten questions and ten follow up questions that they could ask to start conversation using small talk. Follow-up questions are those that they can ask in addition, so the conversation doesn't halt immediately. For instance, they could ask, 'Did you have a nice holiday?' and as a follow up, 'Where did you go?'

Activity 32 Small talk

Appropriate

Not appropriate

Weather 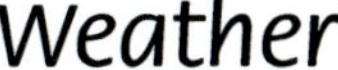	Politics 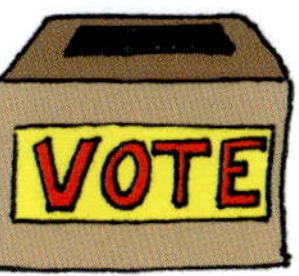
Favourite food 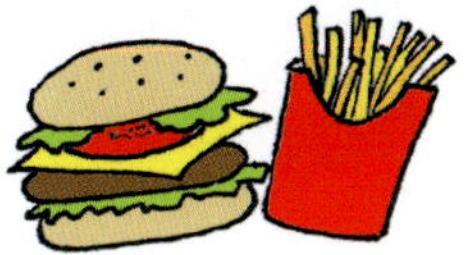	Popular music 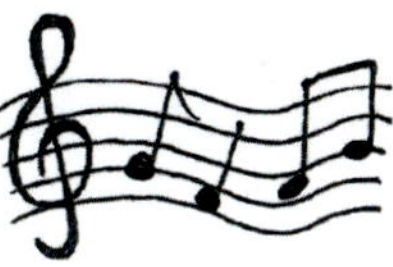
Offensive jokes 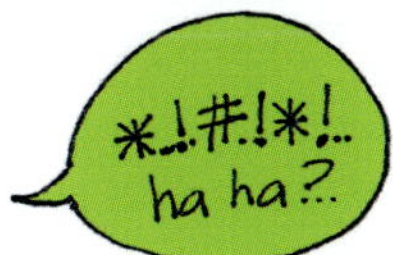	Sickness 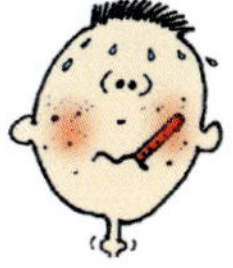
Family 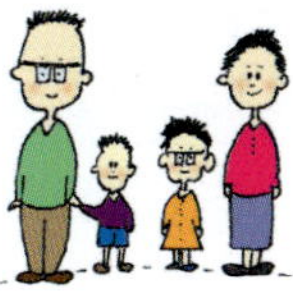	How old someone is 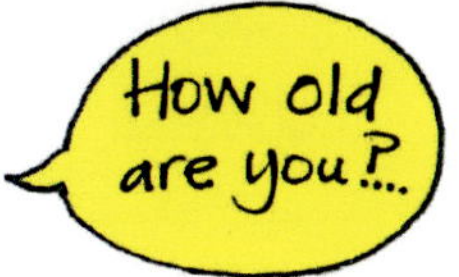

Activity 32 Small talk

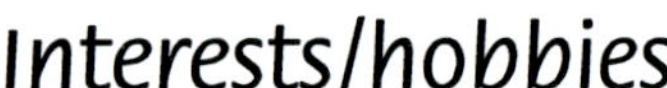
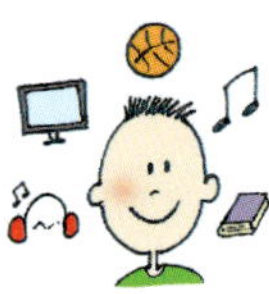

Interests/hobbies

Money
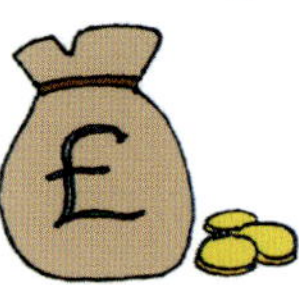

Religion

Popular movies/TV
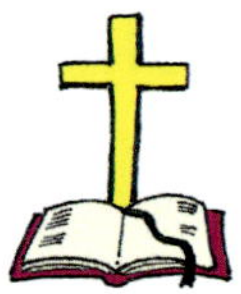
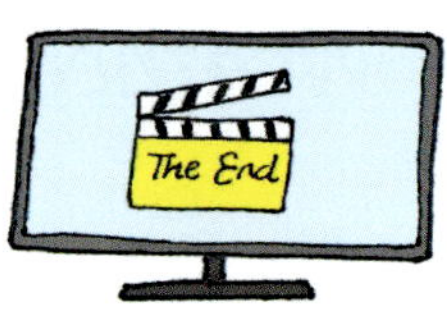

Work

Sports
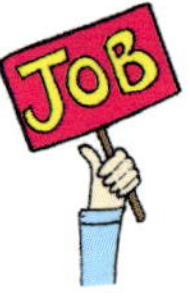
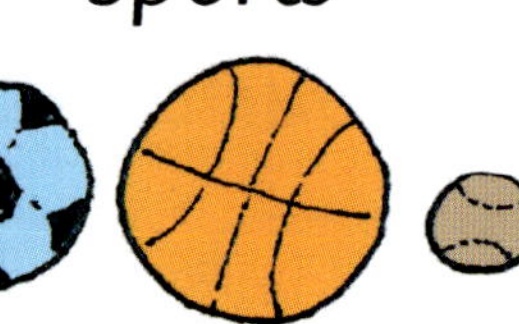

How someone looks

Local news
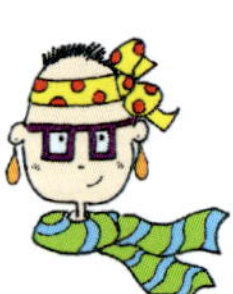
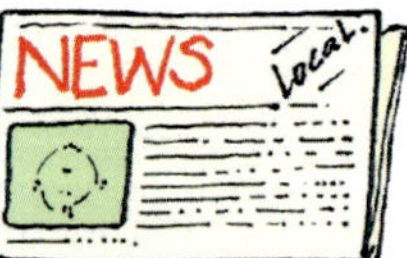

Holidays

Favourite books
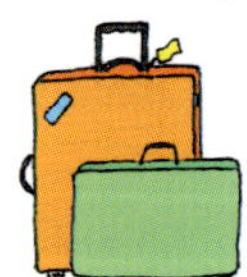
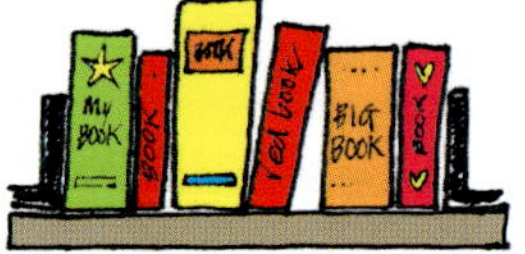

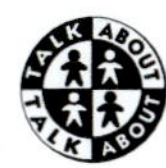
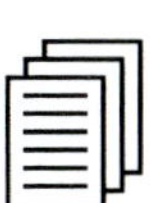

Activity 32 Small talk

Write down or stick in items that are appropriate for small talk:

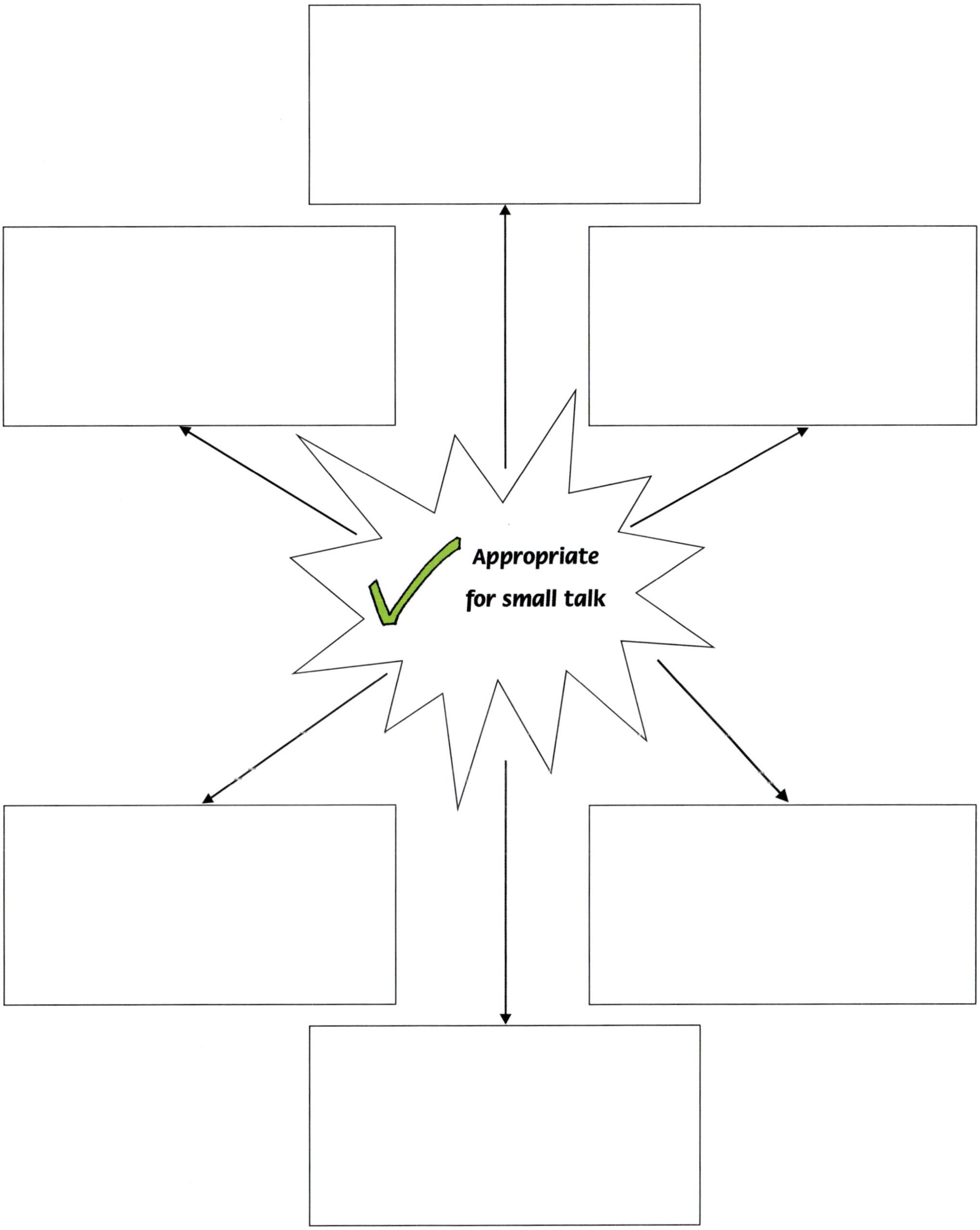

Activity 32 Small talk

Write down or stick in items that are inappropriate for small talk:

Activity 32 Small talk

Conversation starters

Weather:

Question: ....

Follow-up question: ....

Food:

Question: ....

Follow-up question: ....

Music:

Question: ....

Follow-up question: ....

Family:

Question: ....

Follow-up question: ....

Interests/hobbies:

Question: ....

Follow-up question: ....

Activity 32 Small talk

Conversation starters

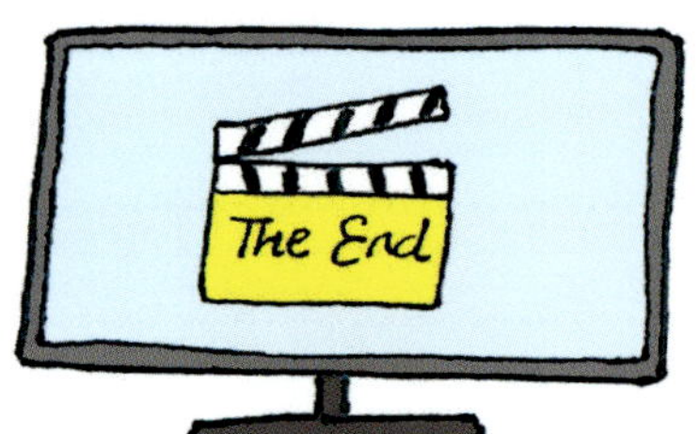

Movies/TV:

Question: ....

Follow-up question: ....

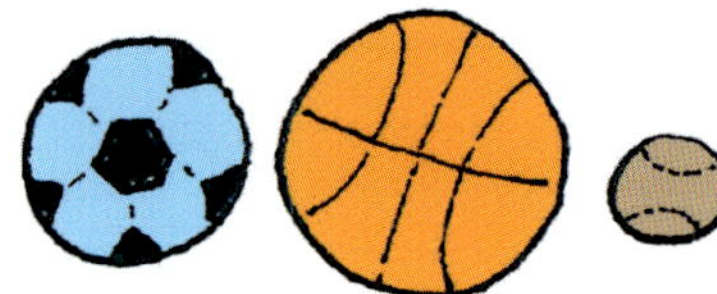

Sports:

Question: ....

Follow-up question: ....

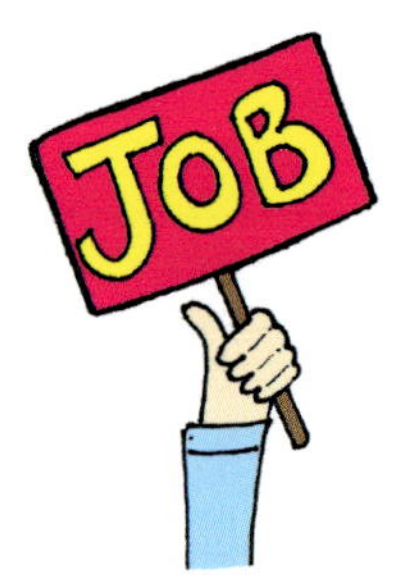

Work:

Question: ....

Follow-up question: ....

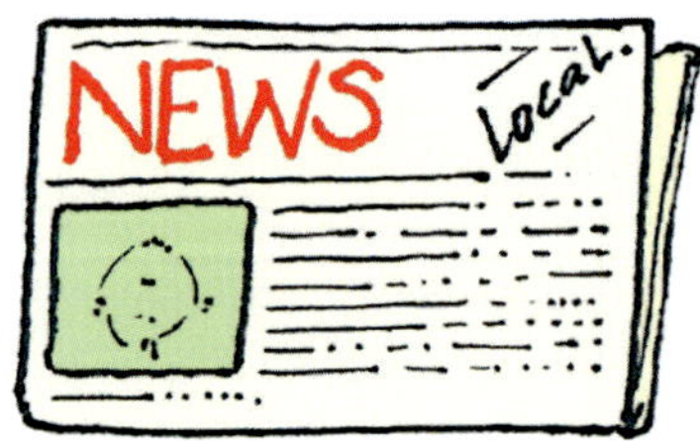

Local news:

Question: ....

Follow-up question: ....

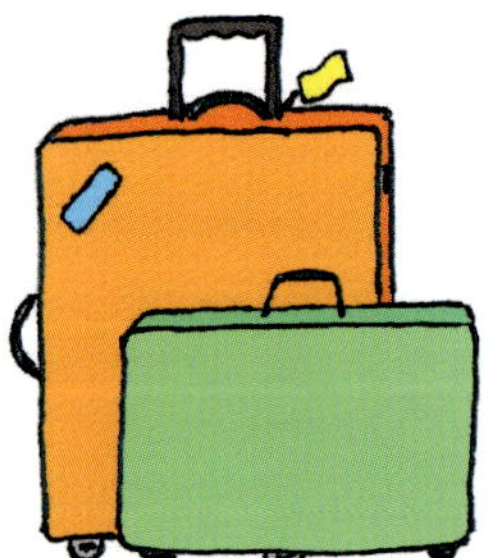

Holidays:

Question: ....

Follow-up question: ....

Activity 33 Dealing with conflict

Preparation

Photocopy and cut up the scenario cards. Photocopy the worksheets.

Instructions

- Introduce the activity by saying that when we work in a team of people, we will sometimes disagree with them. This disagreement might be a small idea or a big argument. We don't always have to like the people we work with to do our job. However, we need to deal with conflict appropriately and responsibly and in a way that resolves the conflict so that a positive working relationship can be restored.

- Place the cards in the middle of the group and ask one group member at a time to pick a card. They can then read out the scenario and decide what would be the best way to approach and resolve the conflict. Positive approaches would be to: stay calm, use good listening skills to ensure you understand what has happened, speak clearly, say what you think and how you feel, and walk away if you feel angry or upset. Approaches that would make the conflict worse include: ignoring the conflict, insulting the person, keeping your feelings about the situation secret, going along with it for an easy life, and getting angry or aggressive.

- This activity can continue until all scenarios have been discussed or all the ideas have been elicited. The group can then discuss why it is important to handle conflict in the workplace.

- The group should then complete the worksheet on dealing with conflict, filling in the box on how to react in a situation.

Activity 33 Dealing with conflict

You and one of your colleagues have never really liked each other. One day, they offer to make everyone a drink except for you.

Someone you work with is constantly late for work and you tell them that they need to be on time. They ignore you for the rest of the day.

You know that one of your colleagues has been lying about how much work they've been doing for a group project. When it comes to the day of the presentation, they're not prepared at all.

One of your colleagues becomes very angry when you disagree with something they've done. They start shouting and pointing their finger at you, blaming you for what's happened.

You were dating one of your colleagues and now you've broken up. You work in different departments but you still see each other every day.

One of your colleagues keeps telling you what to do and is very bossy even though they're not your manager. It makes you really angry and you want to yell at them.

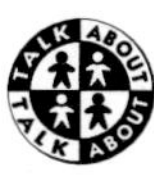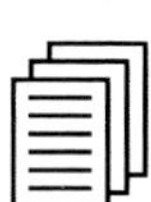

Activity 33 Dealing with conflict

Someone on your team never finishes their work on time and this makes you late to hand in the finished project.

The person you sit next to in the office always asks you questions to see how much you are paid.

Whenever you point out a mistake that one of your colleagues makes, they become very defensive and take the criticism badly.

Someone is gossiping about one of their managers. They say that they wish the manager would leave because then everyone would be happier.
You like the manager and think this is unfair.

The person sitting next to you is jealous of your positive relationship with the manager. They often tell you that they wish they were the manager's favourite.

One of your colleagues never listens to what you say. One day, they miss an important piece of information that you told them about weeks ago, and make the company look bad in front of a customer.

Activity 33 Dealing with conflict

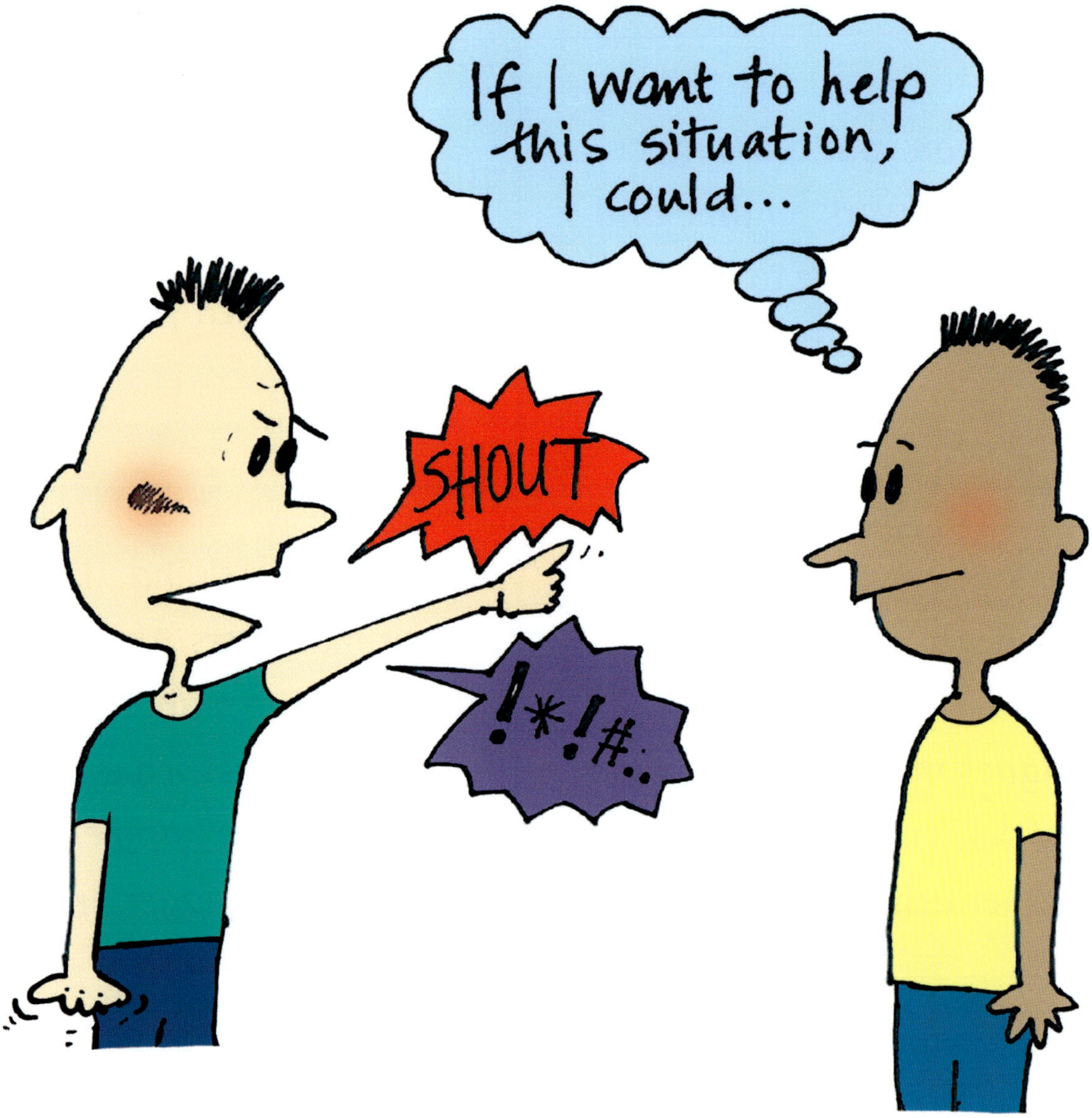

Five things I could do to deal with conflict are:

1. ....

2. ....

3. ....

4. ....

5. ....

Activity 34 Stranded

Preparation

Photocopy and cut out the object labels. Have two large sheets of paper or a whiteboard available to the group. Photocopy the worksheet and provide a copy to each of the group members.

Instructions

- If possible, place the 'Taking'/'Leaving' headings on the whiteboard or one each on the two sheets of paper. Put sticky tack on the back of the object labels and lay them out for the group to see.

- Explain that the group members were travelling on a small boat and sailed through a storm. Their boat has hit a desert island and they are now stranded. The boat is falling apart and will soon sink into the sea, so the group need to determine what they want to save from it. They can choose ten items from the 20 available. Which ones will help them survive the longest? They must give reasons for their answers and the group leaders should encourage debate.

- When the group has decided that they are taking or leaving an item they can stick it under the appropriate heading, but they can also change it later if they need to.

- When completing this activity, the good team-working skills and attributes you should try to elicit include listening, taking turns to ensure that everyone is part of the activity, sharing ideas, taking criticism well, complimenting others on their decisions, how and when to disagree, and compromising. It is important that you identify these when they arise and label them for the group to notice.

- The group may need to decide on who makes the final decision – is it a vague consensus, or will they vote? Will one person have the final decision?

- This activity is only one of many team-building activities available. If you feel that the group would benefit from further team-building, or you feel that there are skills from the list above that would be worth revisiting, you could research some more activities on the internet. Some example team-building games to search for are: Marshmallow Spaghetti Tower, Human Knot, paper plane contests, Minefield, Frostbite and any activities involving the use of Lego.

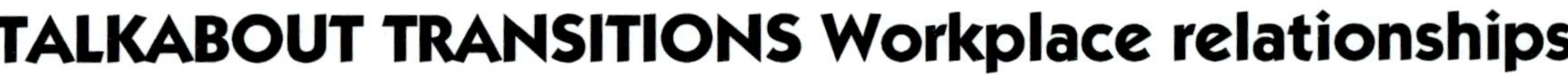

Taking

Leaving

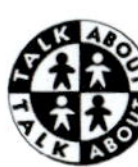
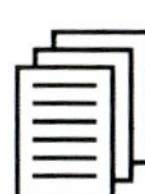

Activity 34 Stranded

Matches

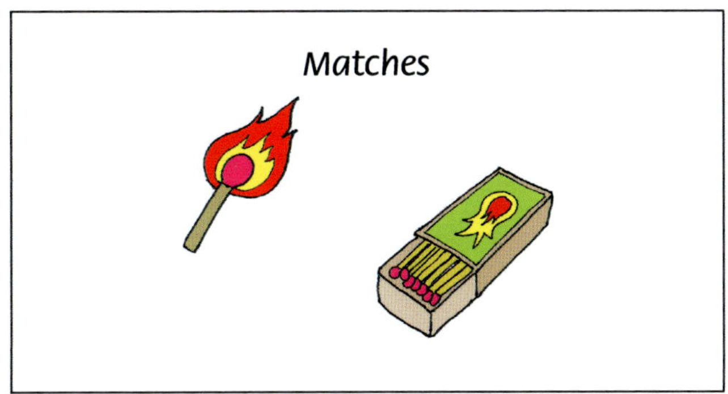

Bottled water

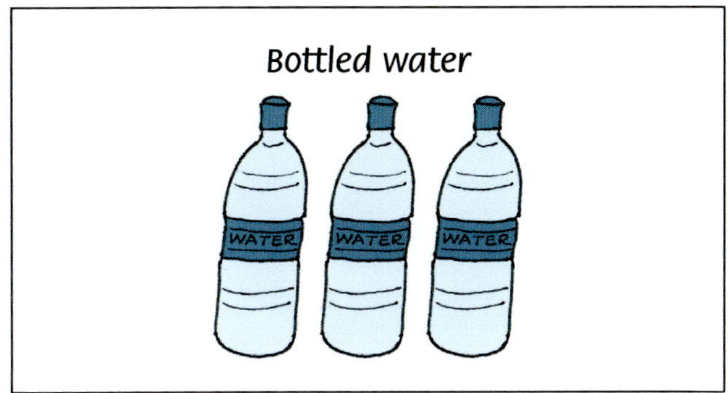

Toolbox

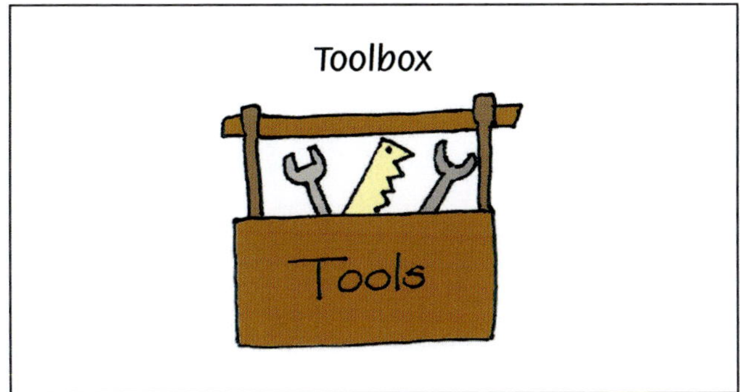

First aid kit

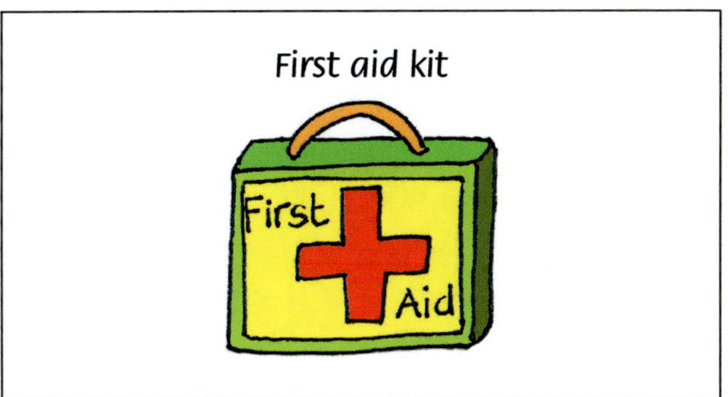

Shovel

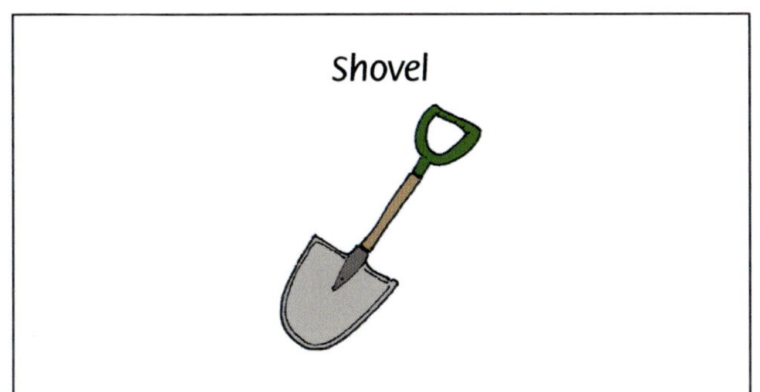

Rope

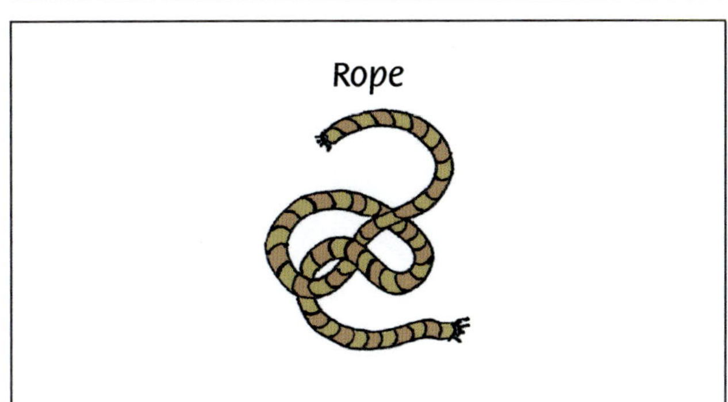

Laptop

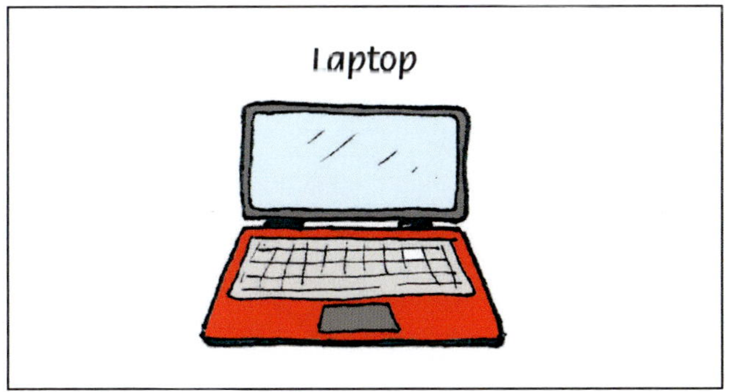

Inflatable raft

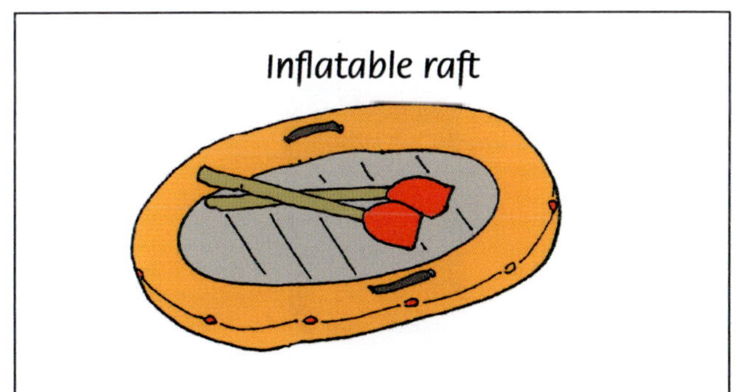

Notebook & pencil

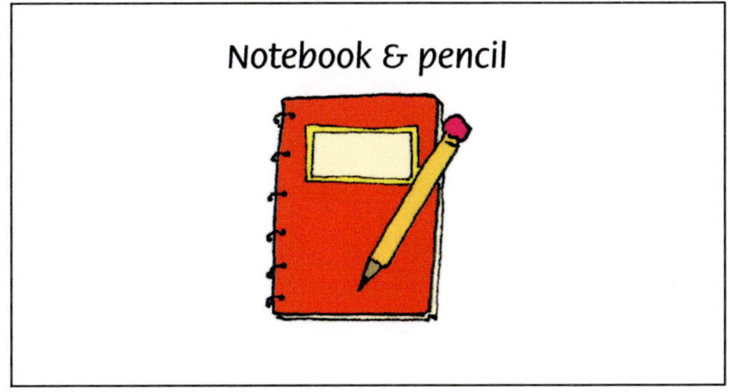

Whistle

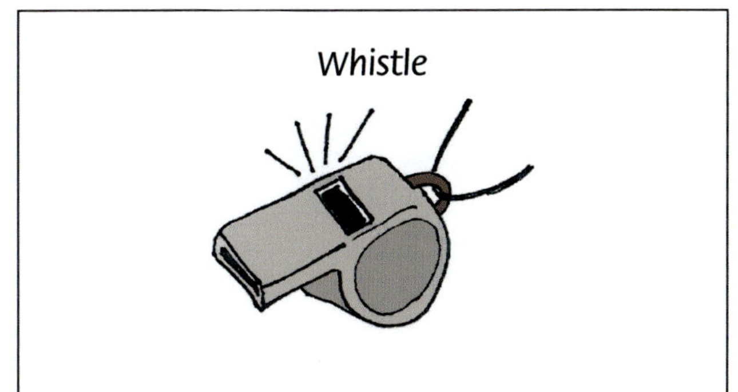

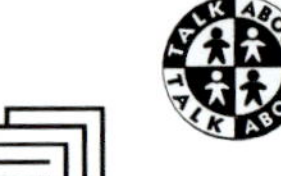

Activity 34 Stranded

Blankets 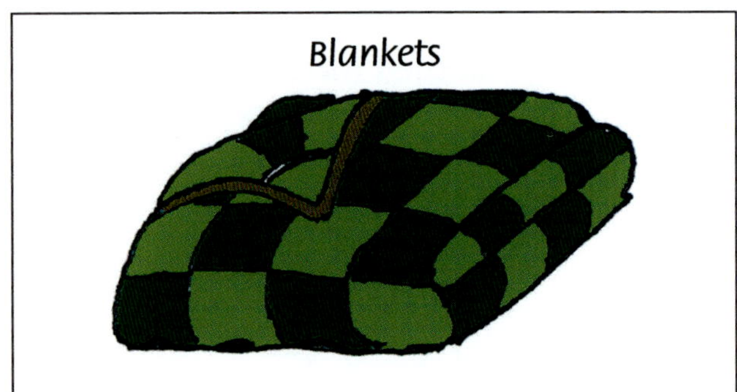	Torch 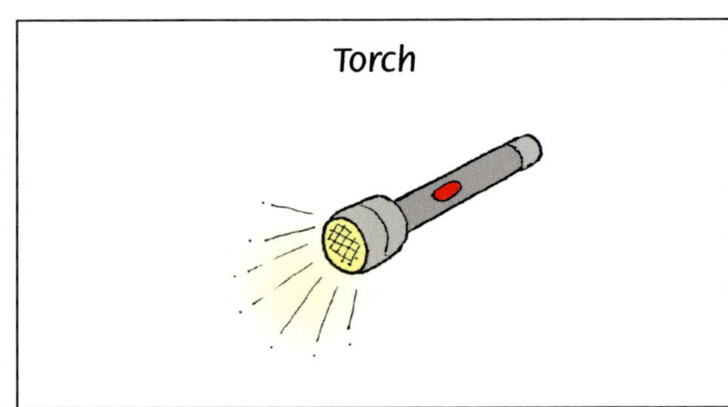
Travel games 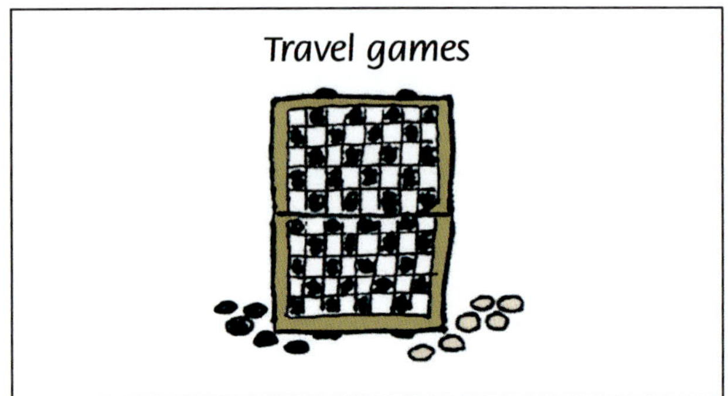	Peanuts 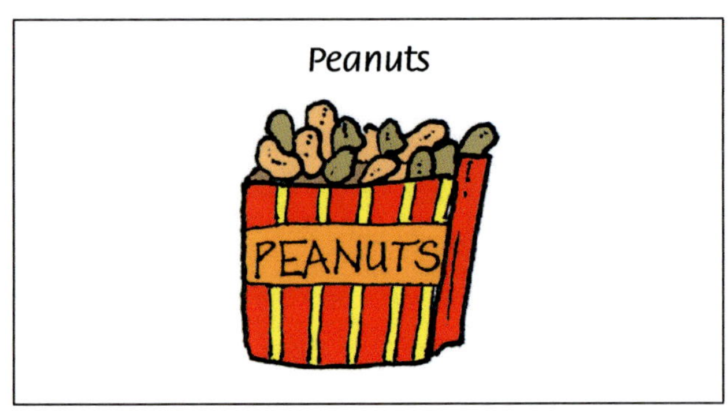
Axe 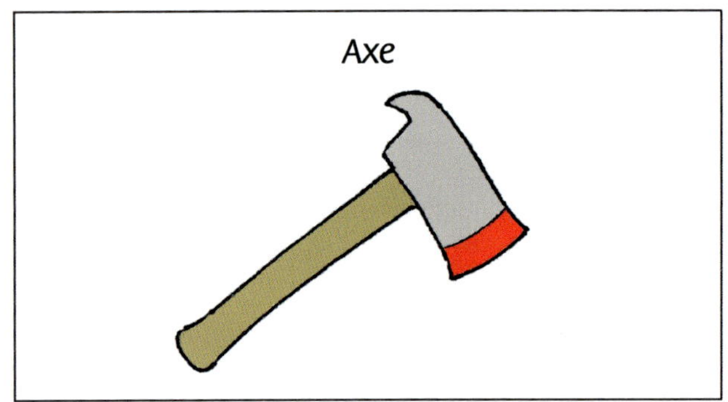	Radio 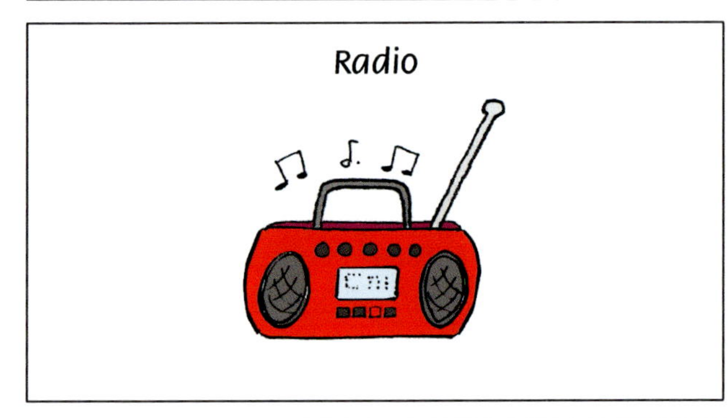
Mobile phone 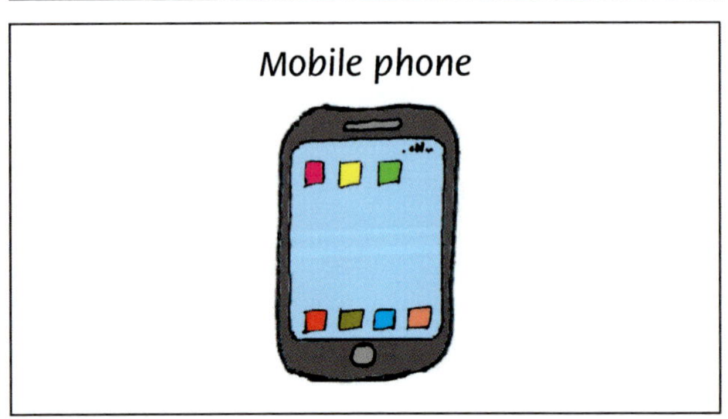	Chocolate bars 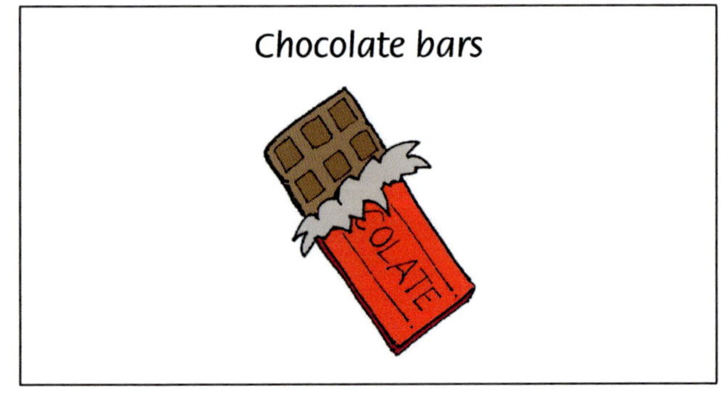
Insect repellent 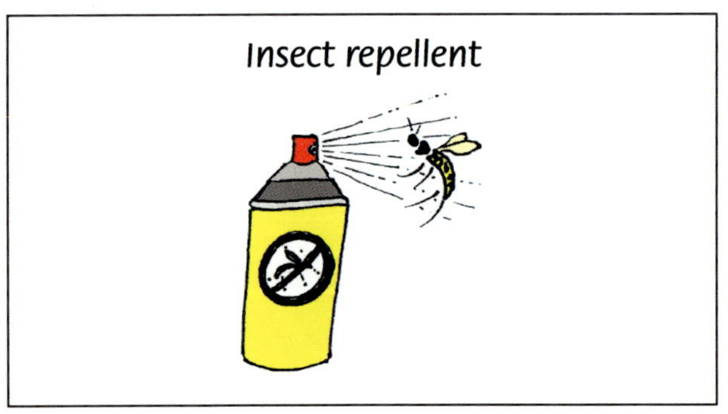	Mirror 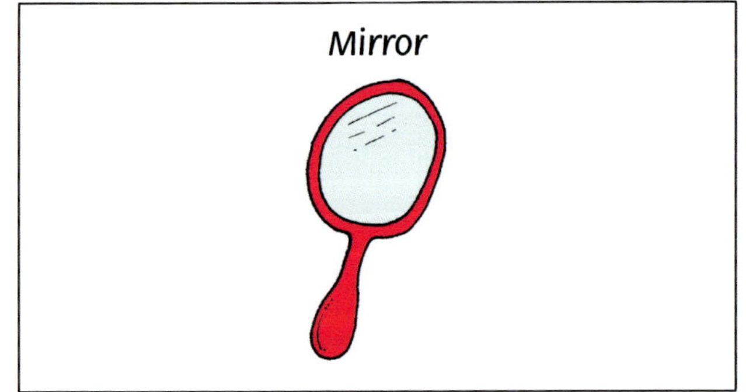

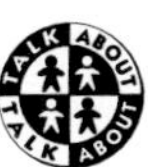
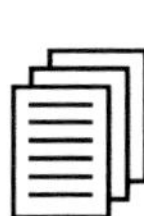

Activity 35 It's a wrap!

This is designed to be the final activity in the whole programme. If you are intending to do the additional problem-solving activities in Topic 6, it is recommended that you carry out this current activity once you have finished those.

Preparation

Photocopy the worksheet.

Instructions

- Before giving each group member a worksheet, ask them to think about the sessions they've completed in the transitions programme. What was their favourite part? What have they learnt? What do they think they could still get better at? Encourage discussion and reflection between the group and ensure that everyone has a turn sharing.

- Give the group members the worksheet and ask them to fill this in. Congratulate them on completing the programme!

Activity 35 It's a wrap!

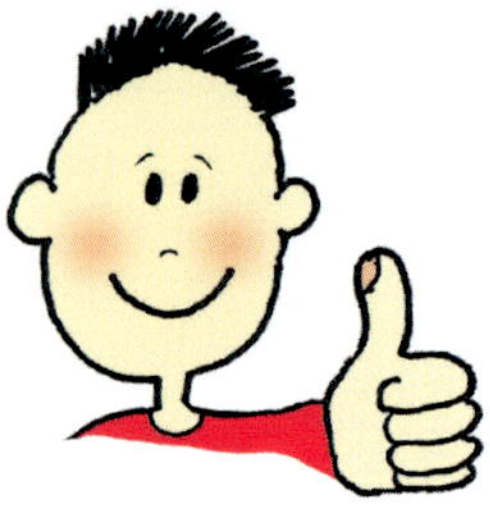

My favourite activity in the transitions group was:

....

....

Three things that I've learnt in the transitions group are:

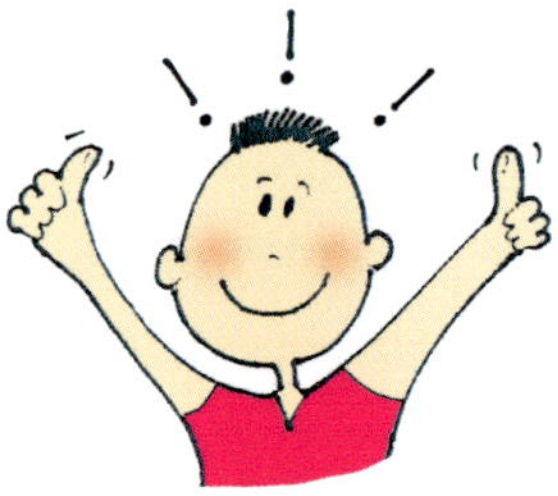

1. ....

....

2. ....

....

3. ....

....

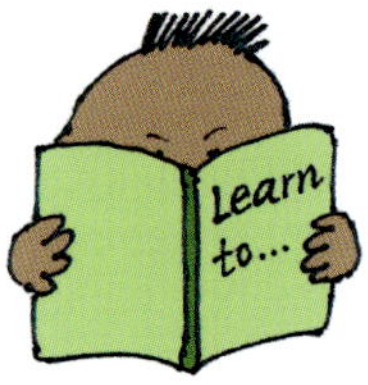

One thing I could still get better at is:

....

....

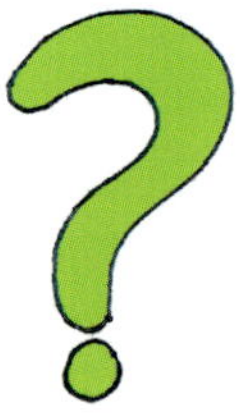

Now the group is finished, I am looking forward to:

....

....

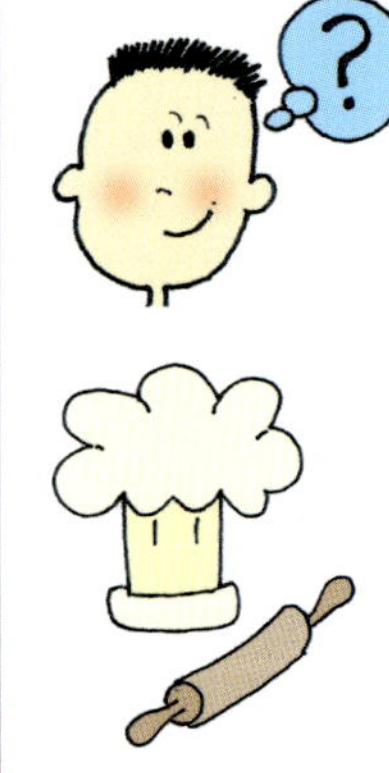

Congratulations!
You have completed
Talkabout Transitions!

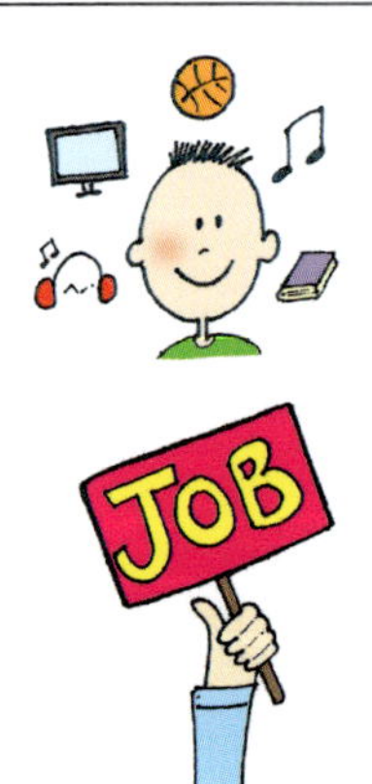

Topic 6 – Problem-solving

Objectives
To develop a range of repeatable and effective strategies to explore and reflect on everyday problems or difficulties.

Timing
This topic is optional but recommended. Many people who experience social skills difficulties also experience difficulties solving problems effectively. It is recommended that a lesson is spent on each one and then the group leaders can revisit these when appropriate to reinforce the different approaches. Alternatively, the group leaders can pick out relevant problem-solving strategies that the group may benefit from at certain times.

Activity	Description
Mindfulness (Activity 36)	The group members carry out an awareness activity and read through a handout on mindfulness. If appropriate, the group leader can then lead a body scan practice.
FACs (Activity 37)	The group are introduced to the FACs framework and use this to solve a problem or difficulty.
Thoughts, feelings and behaviours (Activity 38)	The group are introduced to the thoughts, feelings and behaviours framework and use this to solve a problem or difficulty.
Solutions (Activity 39)	The group are introduced to the solution-focused framework and use this to solve a problem or difficulty.
Time planner (Activity 40)	The group are introduced to the Eisenhower matrix for time management and practise using this to plan their time effectively.
Scenario cards	Each scenario card depicts a problem or difficulty in the workplace or at school/college. These provide a prompt for the group members to access the problem-solving frameworks above.

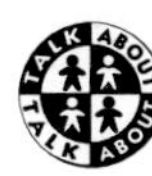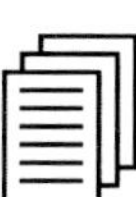

Activity 36 Mindfulness

Preparation

Photocopy the 'Mindfulness awareness countdown' and the 'What is it?' worksheet for each group member. Create a relaxing environment in the room where the group works.

Mindfulness and the body scan meditation isn't for everyone, but it is an exceptional and proactive tool to encourage awareness of the group members' emotional states and allows them to take a step back to see a problem in a different, more objective light.

Instructions

- The aim of this activity is to provide the group members with ways of bringing their attention back to the present moment and accept anxious thoughts.

- Each group member should go through the 'Mindfulness awareness countdown' worksheet and fill in five things they can see, four things they can hear, three things they can feel, two things they can smell and one thing they can taste. This allows the students to shift their focus to what is going on in their body and around them.

- Watch the following videos to see the effect of mindfulness: *Release – https:// vimeo.com/170687659* and *Mindfulness: Youth Voices – https://www.youtube.com/ watch?v=kk7IBwuhXWM*

- Provide the group members with the 'What is it?' handout and discuss the content in the group.

- If the group is relaxed, the group leader should then read through the 'Body scan' script. Once this is finished, reflect on how the group is feeling and what they noticed about the exercise.

Activity 36 Mindful awareness countdown

Write down five things you can see

Write down four things you can hear

Write down three things you can feel

Write down two things you can smell

Write down one thing you can taste

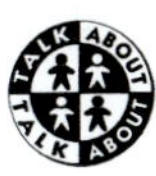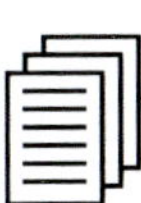

Activity 36 Mindfulness – what is it?

Mindfulness means paying attention to your thoughts, feelings and experiences in the present moment.

Anyone can practise mindfulness and you don't have to change your beliefs.

It originates from Buddhism.

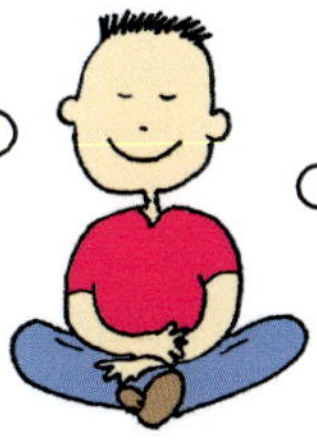

Benefits include having an alert mind, having better self-awareness and becoming less reactive to difficult situations.

There is evidence that mindfulness helps people cope with physical and mental health difficulties.

You can practise it anywhere.

(Apart from when you're asleep!)

We can develop our ability to be mindful by practising it regularly.

Activity 36 Mindfulness – the body scan

> **Read the script through in a relaxed manner.**

Make yourself comfortable. Make sure your back is straight and your feet are flat on the floor. Allow your hands to rest in your lap. Gently close your eyes and take in some long, slow breaths. Breathe in through your nose and feel your stomach and chest expand. Breathe out, feeling the air come out of your nostrils or your mouth. Don't worry if you become distracted at all. Notice this and then bring your attention back to your breath or to the place in the body which I'm talking about.

Notice your feet on the floor, any feeling of your feet in your socks or your shoes, or touching the floor. Notice the pressure and any heat. If you don't notice anything, that's okay too.

Notice your legs, from your calves up to your knees and then your thighs. Move your attention through each part and notice any sensations that might come up. If you feel any discomfort, just observe this and move on.

Bring your attention to your lower back and your stomach area. Notice the breath making the belly expand and decrease in size. You might observe how your clothing feels or some tension in that area. Observe these and let them go.

Move on to your chest area and notice your heartbeat. Feel your chest rise and fall with the breath.

Move your attention to your hands, your fingertips. Move up the arm, through the elbow and up to your shoulders. You might notice differences between your left and your right arm. Let your shoulders relax if they feel tense.

Now, observe your throat, your jaw, your face, the top of your head. Feel the breath in your nostrils or your mouth.

Then notice the whole of your body and take a few more deep breaths. When you feel ready, you may open your eyes.

> **After the body scan is finished, encourage the group members to discuss if they noticed any thoughts or feelings that arose.**

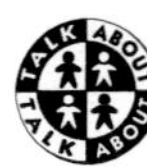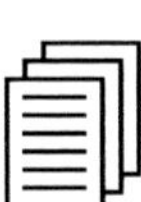

Activity 37 FACs

Preparation

Photocopy the handout and worksheet 'Get your FACs straight'. If appropriate, draw out the structure on a whiteboard or piece of A3 paper and encourage the group members to write the information in the gaps with support.

Instructions

- Either choose a couple of problem scenarios from the problem cards at the end of this chapter or, if appropriate, see if the group members can think of a relevant difficulty in their lives that they would like to tackle with this framework.

- The group leader should go through the handout with the group members, discussing each individual section. FACs stands for **feelings, actions** and **consequences**. This is to introduce the group members to the idea that a situation can affect our feelings, which can affect our actions. These can in turn affect the feelings and behaviours of others and all of this has consequences.

- Once the group members have looked at the handout, encourage them to discuss one of the problem scenarios from the problem cards. Ask them to map the feelings and actions of the characters onto their worksheet.

- As an extension, if they would like to discuss a recent problem that they have had, the leaders should encourage the group to map this real-life situation onto another worksheet.

Activity 37 FACs

Activity 37 Get your FACs straight

Describe the situation (Who was there? Where was it? What happened?)

People, places and events will normally have an effect on our feelings and our behaviours.

Some situations are more difficult for us than others.

FEELING

I felt... Remember that it doesn't matter what emotion we feel, it's

what we do about it that's important.

ACTION

I chose to... What you choose to do will have an immediate impact on

what other people feel and do.

FEELING

They felt... You don't have control over their feelings, but they will be

a result of your actions.

ACTION

They chose to... Their actions will be a result of what they decide to

do about their feelings.

CONSEQUENCES (what happened at the end?)

The consequences of our choices or actions can be positive or negative. It's up to us to make

the right choices.

Could you have done anything differently?

What would change the situation to make a positive outcome?

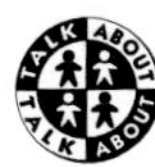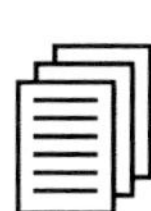

Activity 37 Get your FACs straight

Describe the situation (Who was there? Where was it? What happened?)

FEELING

I felt…

ACTION

I chose to…

FEELING

They felt…

ACTION

They chose to…

CONSEQUENCES (what happened at the end?)

Could you have done anything differently?

Activity 38 Thoughts, feelings and behaviours

Preparation

Photocopy the handout and worksheet 'Thoughts, feelings and behaviours'. If appropriate, draw out the structure on a whiteboard or piece of A3 paper and encourage the group members to write the information in the gaps with support from the group.

Instructions

- Either choose a couple of problem scenarios from the problem cards at the end of this chapter or, if appropriate, see if the group members can think of a relevant difficulty in their lives that they would like to tackle with this framework.

- Work through the handout with the group members, discussing each individual section. This is to introduce the group members to the idea that in a certain situation there are lots of factors that might influence our thoughts and feelings. These can in turn affect our behaviours and there will be consequences of this.

- Once the group members have looked at the handout, encourage them to discuss one of the problem scenarios from the problem cards. Ask them to map the internal and external factors involved in the situation, and then the thoughts and feelings, behaviours and consequences of the characters onto their worksheet.

- As an extension, if they would like to discuss a recent problem that they have had, the leaders should encourage the group to map this real-life situation onto another worksheet.

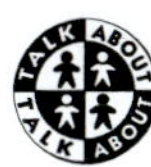
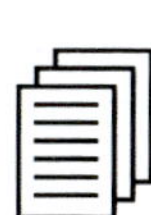

Activity 38 Thoughts, feelings and behaviours

Situation: ....

....

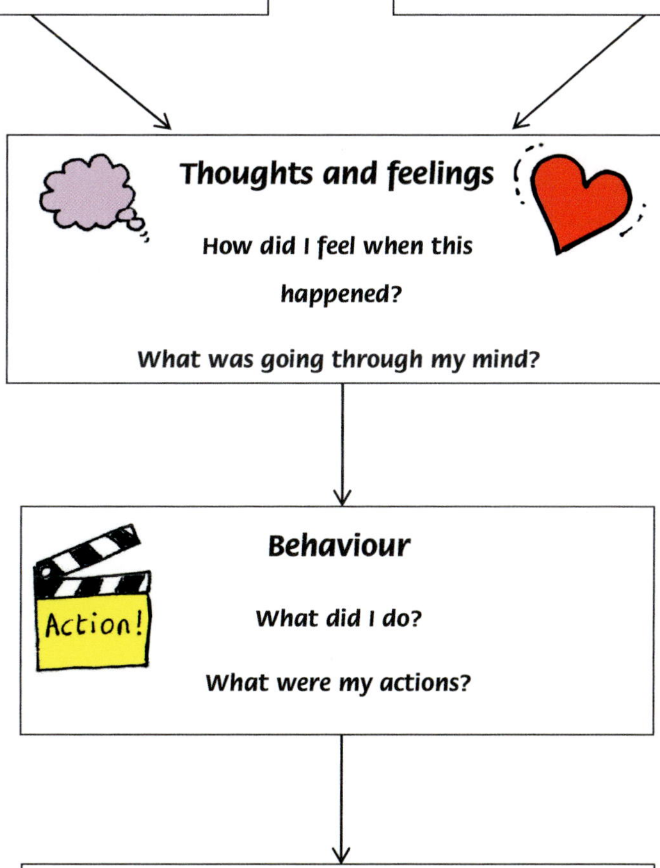

Activity 38 Thoughts, feelings and behaviours

Situation: ....

....

<table>
<tr><td>External factors</td><td>Internal factors</td></tr>
</table>

Thoughts and feelings

Behaviour

Consequences

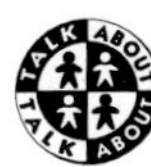
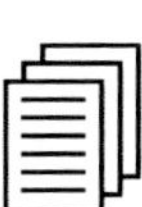

Activity 39 Solutions

Preparation

Provide the group members with the worksheet 'Solutions'. If appropriate, draw out the structure on a whiteboard or piece of A3 paper and encourage the group members to write the information in the gaps with support from the group.

Instructions

- Either choose a couple of problem scenarios from the problem cards at the end of this chapter or, if appropriate, see if the group members can think of a relevant difficulty in their lives that they would like to tackle with this framework.

- The group leaders should go through an example of one situation, encouraging the group to come up with five different solutions – it doesn't matter if they're silly ideas! When there are five solutions written down in the bubbles, the group should think about what the consequences of each one would be and rate these out of ten. This will leave the group with one or two options which are the best based on their ratings.

- Once this has been done, provide them with some problems/scenario cards and see how many appropriate solutions they can come up with on their worksheet.

- As an extension, if they would like to discuss a recent problem that they have had, the leaders should encourage the group to map this real-life situation onto another worksheet.

Activity 39 Solutions

Situation (write down a short description of the situation/problem):

In the bubbles below, write down different solutions to the above situation. Think about the consequence of each solution and write this down in the box underneath. Then mark how useful each consequence is out of ten.

Consequence: /10

Consequence: /10

Consequence: /10

Consequence: /10

Consequence: /10

What is the best solution?

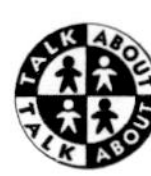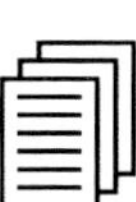

Activity 40 Time planner

Preparation

Provide the group members with the handout and worksheet 'Time matrix'.

Instructions

- The group leaders should go through the examples on the Eisenhower matrix worksheet. This is a time-management tool that the group members can use to prioritise what is important and what is urgent.

- See if the group members can use the worksheet to prioritise the things they need to do for school, college, work or tasks for life on their own matrix. Also see if they can spot tasks which are unimportant and can wait.

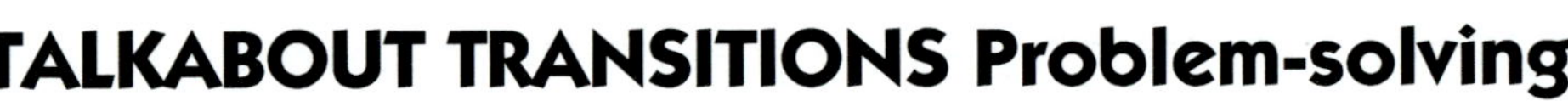
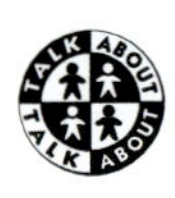
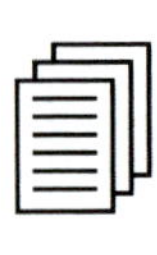

Activity 40 Time planner

	URGENT	NON-URGENT
IMPORTANT	**1. Do it now** These are tasks which are important to your school life, future career or home life. They must be done today or as soon as possible this week. You could set a timer to complete these tasks. These could be things like: • Homework that's due tomorrow • Paying urgent bills • Replacing your car headlight before it has its MOT	**2. Plan it** These are important tasks for your school, life and future career, but aren't as urgent as the first box. This is the most important box as it allows you to plan things in reasonable time, reduce stress and contribute to your long-term goals. You should write a time to do these tasks in your diary or calendar, things like: • Go to the gym again • Researching your coursework for English
NOT IMPORTANT	**3. Delegate it** These are tasks which might look important but aren't really. You might also be able to ask someone else to do these or support someone to come up with ideas to their own problems. You can keep track of them by phone or email. They might be: • Your friend urgently needs your help with homework • Checking your phone for text messages	**4. Ignore it** These tasks are unimportant for what you want to achieve in education, work and life. You should ignore them if you have urgent or important work. If you don't have anything important to do, then you can enjoy them! These might be: • Watching TV • Playing video games • Browsing the internet aimlessly

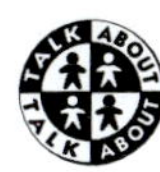
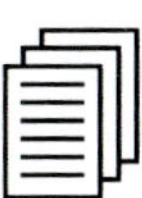

Activity 40 Time planner

	URGENT	NON-URGENT
IMPORTANT	1. Do it now	2. Plan it
NOT IMPORTANT	3. Delegate it	4. Ignore it

Scenario cards

These are some possible examples to use in the groups for the problem-solving frameworks. Adapt them as necessary or use as inspiration for new ones.

One of your friends was talking throughout your maths lesson and hasn't done their work. They've asked you if they can copy your work. They did the same thing last week as well.	You told one of your friends a secret and they promised they wouldn't say anything to anyone. You overheard someone talking about your secret in the hallway today.
One of your friends is bullying a person in your class. They keep mocking them when they try to talk and push them around in the cafeteria. They also keep texting them with nasty messages and laughing about it.	You are having an argument with one of your friends about smoking. You think that they shouldn't smoke. They become angry and storm away.
You are worried about one of your friends. They recently said that they were feeling depressed. Now they won't come out shopping with you and are not coming into college.	You called one of your friends a name yesterday and this made them upset. Now they are ignoring you.

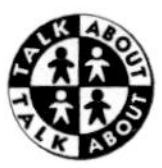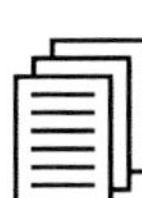

Scenario cards

<table>
<tr>
<td>You meet up with one of your friends to play football and they are racist about someone in your class.</td>
<td>One of your best friends is at your birthday party but you can tell they feel uncomfortable. They are standing by themselves and not really talking to anyone.</td>
</tr>
<tr>
<td>You received your exam results and did well. Your friend didn't do as well as they thought and aren't talking to you anymore. You think they might be jealous.</td>
<td>You get a job which you thought you'd really like. However, you have worked there for a week and you don't seem to be doing the job you applied for.</td>
</tr>
<tr>
<td>You have worked hard on a project at work, but it's gone past the deadline and you haven't finished it. Your manager is disappointed.</td>
<td>One of your colleagues keeps asking for your help on their projects but it means that now you haven't done any of your own work.</td>
</tr>
</table>

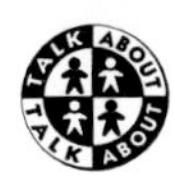

References

Clark, H. B. & Unruh, D. K. (2009). *Transition of Youth and Young Adults with Emotional or Behavioural Difficulties*, Maryland: Paul H. Brookes Publishing.

Waddell, G. & Burton, K. (2006). *Is Work Good for Your Health and Well-being? An Independent Review*. Norwich: Department for Work and Pensions.

National Mental Health Development Unit (2010). *Factfile 1: Mental Health and Employment*. London: Department of Health.

Department for Business, Innovation and Skills (2013). *The Impact of Further Education Learning*. London: Department for Business, Innovation and Skills.

Broadhurst, S., Yates, K. & Mullen, B. (2012). 'An evaluation of the My Way transition programme'. *Tizard Learning Disability Review*, Vol. 17, Issue 3, pp.124–134, https://doi.org/10.1108/13595471211240960

Robles, M. (2012). 'Executive perceptions of the top 10 soft skills needed in today's workplace'. *Business Communication Quarterly*, Vol. 75, Issue 4, pp. 453–465.

Schulz, B. (2008). 'The Importance of Soft Skills: Education beyond academic knowledge'. *Journal of Language and Communication*, June, pp. 146–154.

Nickson, D., Warhurst, C., Commander, J., Hurrell, S. A. & Cullen, A. (2011). 'Soft skills and employability: Evidence from UK retail'. *Economic and Industrial Democracy*, Vol. 33, Issue 1, pp. 65–84. Originally published online 9 December 2011.

"Release" (2016). Vimeo video, added by wavecrest films [Online]. Available at https://vimeo.com/170687659

Mindfulness: Youth Voices (2013). Youtube video, added by KeltyMentalHealth [Online]. Available at https://www.youtube.com/watch?v=kk7IBwuhXWM

TALKABOUT TRANSITIONS Evaluation form

Evaluation form

Group: .... Date: ....

Session number: ....

Group members present: ....

	Plan	Evaluation
Starter activity		
Main activities		
Finishing activity		

Completed by: ....

Index